SAVING MY SONS

SAVING MY SONS

A Journey with Autism

Ilana Gerschlowitz with Marion Scher

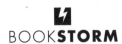

BOOK**STORM**

ISBN: 978-1-928257-64-6
e-ISBN: 978-1-928257-65-3

First edition, first impression 2019

Published by Bookstorm (Pty) Ltd
PO Box 4532
Northcliff 2115
Johannesburg
South Africa
www.bookstorm.co.za

Edited by Isabelle Delvare
Proofread by Wesley Thompson
Cover design by publicide
Book design and typesetting by Triple M Design
Printed by Pinetown Press, Pinetown

This book is dedicated to our eldest son David,
who has taught us patience, perseverance, dedication and
how to be courageous. Above all, he has allowed us to learn the
most important lesson in life –
to see through the superficial to what truly matters.

CONTENTS

ACKNOWLEDGEMENTS

This book and the work we do at The Star Academy would not have been possible without the massive contributions made by my colleagues Jenna White, Reinette Weideman, Carmen du Plooy, Cayla Strauss and Phillip Viljoen, and all the instructors who have told their stories within these pages. There would have been no story without Dr Doreen Granpeesheh and her team at CARD, or without the late Dr Jeff Bradstreet. Other important contributions came from Dr Marco Ruggiero. Thank you also to Advocate Jeremy Goldstone for his invaluable legal input.

Thank you, Marion Scher, for making my words come alive – without you this book would never have happened. Thanks also to the team at Bookstorm: Louise, Russell, Nicola and Danielle.

To Bernie Sher – our mentor and the reason we never left South Africa – thank you for helping to establish The Star Academy and saving countless families such as ours.

We acknowledge our sons Eli and Aaron. Eli, you have been an incredible brother – and so patient with us when it seems as though there is no world outside autism. Aaron, you have brought light into our dark world and continue to delight us every day. We are truly blessed to have you as sons.

Most importantly, I salute my husband Martin for being an incredible husband and father. There are no words to explain the impact of your support and contribution in raising our children; and in changing the course of autism in South Africa by establishing and helping to run The Star Academy.

Finally, to David, the bravest of sons. You have had to work so hard to achieve what others take for granted, and have put up a tremendous fight to overcome your daily challenges. Your battleground has laid the foundation for the success, healing and recovery of countless children on the African continent, including your brother Aaron.

Ilana Gerschlowitz
Johannesburg

FOREWORD

When I first met Ilana, I was immediately struck by her warm heart, positive energy and incredible ability to multitask. She had her hands full, to say the least – she was in the midst of setting up a huge conference, had two young boys to care for, and surely had a million worries. Nevertheless, she had arranged to have a big basket of snacks waiting for me in my hotel room, organised an assistant to be at my beck and call, and scheduled numerous activities to keep my children and I entertained while we were in South Africa. Over the years, I have come to realise that her warmth, caring manner and incredible optimism are a genuine part of her personality. The loving Ilana I met so many years ago has only become stronger by overcoming the obstacles she has faced – and she has certainly faced more than most do in a lifetime.

Parenting a child with autism is a profoundly challenging experience. I have had the privilege of working with hundreds of families over the years and I am continually amazed to see how parents fight for their children, despite the fear and grief they experience. Every parent has a unique and interesting story to tell. Many share a common theme. They worry about their child's future, always wondering: Will my child ever be able to live an independent life, a happy life, a fulfilling life? Many parents face sleepless nights trying to give meaning to the heart-wrenching cries of their child. Many have embarrassing moments in public when their child has a meltdown or a well-meaning stranger tries to tell them how to be a better parent. But few parents can tell the story Ilana tells. Few parents have a child with such severe physical illnesses as David's and fewer still have to face autism twice. Ilana's story sends a powerful message to all parents and professionals in the world of autism: If you want to help a child with autism, discard your biases and preconceptions and beyond all else, never, ever give up. This book demonstrates the value of a parent's persistence, determination and hope.

Over the years, I have lived through the journey of fear, pain and sadness with many families. I have felt the parents' loss of hope deeply in my heart and it is that pain that motivates me to keep looking for answers to guide them as they strive to help their children. I am in awe of the parents of the children I treat. I learn from their strength every day and admire their never-ending determination. As religious leader James Faust once said, 'The depth of the love of parents for their children cannot be measured. It is like no other relationship. It exceeds concern for life itself. The love of a parent for a child is continuous and transcends heartbreak and disappointment.'

As Ilana describes all too well, the experience of having a child with autism begins with a shattering of all hopes. The dreams you have for your child are ripped away in an instant and the challenging behaviours that take over your life are, in a way, your test of survival. You either survive and persist as Ilana did, or you enter a dark state of depression and anxiety which becomes your new normal.

When your child is as severely ill as David was, it is a great challenge to survive. Every parent knows that the sound of your child's cries and the sight of your child's tears are heartbreaking. But not knowing what causes your child's sadness and frustration is devastating. As Ilana explains so well, the parent of the autistic child learns to read their child's every emotion. When David couldn't communicate his fears, his pains or even his needs, it was Ilana who interpreted for him. And when even she couldn't determine the cause of his anguish, watching him scream and realising that he was inconsolable despite their best efforts was more than most parents could imagine. For so many years, Ilana and Martin learnt to cope with what seems unimaginable to the rest of us.

While we have learnt a great deal about autism over the past four decades, we still know very little about its aetiology and we continue to search for answers in treatment. Autism is defined by its symptoms. While the spectrum of autism is wide, all children on the spectrum experience some level of difficulty in communication and in social behaviour.

Children on the spectrum of autism range from having no language at all, being completely isolated and unable to interact with others, to being very adept at speech and only lacking in the social aspects of communication. When a child is first diagnosed with autism, it's difficult, if not impossible, to predict where on the spectrum the child will fall. In fact, the child's full capabilities may not become evident until he or she is much older. Unfortunately, waiting to start treatment can lead to a disastrous outcome as the window of opportunity for learning is at its peak before the age of seven. As such, the most successful interventions – Applied Behavioural Analysis (ABA), in particular – result in the most positive outcome when carried out in the earliest stages of a child's life, ideally as early as age two.

ABA can now be considered a scientifically validated pedagogical approach that has been time-tested and repeatedly proven to be effective throughout the lifetime of individuals with autism and other learning disabilities.

Some parents feel autism defines their child and they prefer to accept it rather than try to change it. I urge those parents to consider this intervention to be simply a tool they can use to help their children reduce the challenging behaviours that keep them isolated from society, and strengthen the skills they need to more successfully interact with those around them.

Other parents, like Ilana, continuously search for treatments that will help their child cope, as they believe that adapting to societal norms is an inevitable requirement of life. For many years, I have guided parents of children with autism. I have urged them to keep an open mind and to find treatments for each aspect of their child's autism. No two children with autism are the same. As we see through Ilana's eyes, David and Aaron, both diagnosed with autism, had very different symptoms, fell on extreme opposite poles of the spectrum of autism, and had very different outcomes. Yet both boys benefited from ABA.

It has always been my belief that autism is a whole-body illness. When a child is physically ill, as David was, treating the illness becomes a priority. In fact, unless those physical illnesses are treated, it becomes difficult, if not impossible, to apply behavioural interventions at all. Intensive behavioural interventions such as ABA can only succeed if the child is healthy enough to receive them. An ill child – one who does not sleep or may be in pain – cannot learn, and any attempts to force instruction can easily become aversive.

Because of this, Ilana walked two very different paths with David and Aaron. David required constant and ongoing medical treatments and much of the hardship of his journey focused on keeping his medical symptoms under control. Unfortunately, this reduced the benefit he gained from ABA. Only a percentage of his time did he feel well enough to actually learn from ABA. But when he did learn, he grabbed on to his knowledge and used it with great functionality. On the other hand, Aaron, who had few physical illnesses, and who benefited from his parents' prior experiences, soaked up his ABA teaching and demonstrated the most positive outcome possible: recovery. Aaron no longer requires support, is fully integrated in a typical school, and has become indistinguishable from his peers.

Despite the many times that I have shared in the joys of – and experienced the anguish of – the families I work with, reading this book took me to a different level. While I was present during some of the struggles Ilana describes with David, I never fully grasped the enormity of pain experienced by the whole family. Their journey was much more difficult than even I had imagined.

David's strength and persistence has also been a lesson for all of us. Often in life, we encounter difficulties that shake us. Few take these difficult moments and turn them into opportunities to help others. As we read in the book, early in David's development, Ilana and Martin took charge of a school. They hired staff and worked closely with us to train all of their employees to gain board certification in the delivery and design of behaviour analytic programmes. Through their schools, they have helped hundreds of other children. They have supported hundreds of parents through the most difficult times of their lives and have helped many children reach levels of functioning they would never have otherwise achieved.

In this book, Ilana has shared intimate details of her family's journey through autism. You will read of joy and achievement, sadness and pain. But in the end, I am certain you will walk away in awe of the strength of parents of children with autism. If you are one such parent yourself, read this book and let hope and determination take the place of guilt and fear.

Dr Doreen Granpeesheh
Founder and CEO, Center for Autism and Related Disorders
California, USA

PREFACE

When you become a journalist and even more an investigative feature writer, you quickly learn that the story comes first and your own emotions last. When you know you're going into an emotionally difficult story, interviewing the very people whose lives have been irrevocably touched by hardship and trauma, you have to keep a professional distance.

When I first met Ilana Gerschlowitz and heard her story, I knew this wouldn't be so easy. What I didn't expect was how this amazing woman's story would touch me in a way no other had in my long career.

As each chapter unfolded, my awe and admiration for Ilana and Martin grew. Just as I thought, 'How much more could a family take?' I learnt just how much ...

Perhaps the hardest part of writing this book with Ilana was simply finding the time between running The Star Academy and being a mother of three boys – but somehow we managed to get three or four hours a week together for around 18 months. I would often receive emails form Ilana at 4 am bursting with ideas. I learnt that this was Ilana's premium writing time and when you realise just what she crams into a day, you understand the mammoth task this book was for her.

To co-write a book such as this, it's vital that the person whose story you're telling is completely open with you, holding nothing back, so you can bring their feelings and emotions to the page. This is what makes this story stand apart. Ilana, Martin and Eli were completely open in telling their stories. This was sometimes cathartic for them, and often painful.

Although there are many very moving parts to this tale, there are also so many uplifting moments – none more than Aaron's story. Getting to know this wonderful, vibrant six-year-old has been another bonus of writing this book.

What also made my job so much easier was the enthusiasm so many autism experts from around the world had in co-operating on this project. The relentless Ilana, in her search for answers, has found the finest experts in the world to unravel the mystery that is autism.

Now, seeing this book in print, I'm excited at the prospect of so many people finding the answers that they've been seeking for so long. You only have to sit in Ilana's office for an hour or two listening to her staff fielding calls from desperate parents to know this book will make a difference. What an honour and a privilege to have been part of this project.

Marion Scher
Johannesburg

PROLOGUE

How do you start explaining an illness that few really understand? Mention the word 'autism' and you'll get a whole range of different opinions. Even after 15 years of searching and many discoveries later, our family is still unravelling the mystery. This book invites you to join us on an intriguing journey through many twists and turns (and even mazes!) – in other words, the journey that eventually led us out of the stranglehold of autism. By sharing our personal experiences about reaching out to and extracting our son David from the condition that trapped him, we touch on what we learnt about treating autism and how to create a new 'normal'.

In telling our story, we share what we have gone through and the details of David's diagnosis and treatment, passing on our first-hand knowledge and experience of what it means to be the parents of a child with autism. What we've learnt over the years is that in autism there is only one constant – which is that each child is different. As the saying goes: 'If you've met one individual with autism, you've met one individual with autism.'

This book is not just about David's story. It's about a family with three beautiful boys, and our journey into the world of autism. This is our story of staggering heartbreak, searing honesty and, most importantly, monumental victories.

CHAPTER ONE

THE PERFECT LIFE

Growing up and meeting the love of our lives

ILANA'S STORY

Having grown up on a farm near Kestell in the Free State, I have fond memories of waking up to the smell of my mother's delicious farm breakfasts. As a small child I loved every moment of running around barefoot in the dusty wheat fields. You'd often find me in the stable feeding the calves or taking care of one of the abandoned lambs we'd picked up in a field. I learnt to drive and park a tractor when I was ten years old, and would climb the water tanks and wheat silos and sit on the highest platforms to do my homework.

As we couldn't always get everything we needed in Kestell, we'd often make the three-hour drive from the farm to Johannesburg. As I grew older, and especially during my teenage years, I longed to live in the city and dreamt about studying and working there one day. It seemed so glamorous and exciting!

My mother, who had grown up in a traditional, religious Jewish home, made sure we kept kosher and the traditional laws, even though the logistics involved were difficult.

At the end of December 1992, at the age of 17, I completed my matric in Afrikaans although my home language was English. I moved to Johannesburg to study a commerce degree through the University of South Africa, and shared an apartment with my older brother who'd already been living in Johannesburg for some time. Finally, I'd moved to the big city to live the life I'd dreamt about.

My first year in Johannesburg was daunting and I felt overwhelmed by having to juggle a social life with my studies. In an attempt to make friends, I decided to join a group of students who were going on a weekend away. It was there I met Martin for the first time. I fell in love instantly with this tall, dark and handsome boy, who in no time managed to sweep me off my feet and steal my heart forever.

After completing my undergraduate commerce degree, I went on to do a law degree through Wits University. I finished it in 1998 and started my career as an attorney in 1999. After two years of articles at a prominent law firm in Johannesburg, I continued to specialise in labour law. My perfectly mapped-out life was firmly on track.

Martin's story

As a little boy I grew up on the friendly streets of Port Elizabeth in the Eastern Cape. My parents raised me in a traditional, religious Jewish home. At one stage my grandmother, her sister, my mother and her sister and our family all lived on the same street. Sport was my life and I was happiest when I was holding or kicking a ball. I took part in sport before, during and after school.

It was a carefree childhood in a quiet suburb where we rode our bikes in the streets and walked around without a care in the world. When my younger brother and I played tennis in the street, we'd put up a makeshift net that spanned the entire road. Every so often a car would come past, and it would have to stop while we lowered the net so it could pass.

When I was 14, my parents made the decision to move to Johannesburg. The big city was overwhelming for me. In PE I was a big fish in a little pond, but in Johannesburg no one knew me and I battled to get selected into the top sports teams.

I completed matric in 1990 and enrolled at Wits University to become a chartered accountant. I'd set my sights on becoming a successful business man. While at university I was eager to earn my own income and my uncle helped me set up a business. I'd buy CDs from a wholesaler and sell them to restaurants and stores – anybody who'd invite me into their store.

Every year some Jewish students got together for a weekend away and it was there I first laid eyes on Ilana. What drew me to her was her pretty smile and carefree disposition. She seemed so happy, and smiled almost all the time. After our first date, I knew I'd met the woman I'd marry. I'd never before met a girl who cleaned her plate on a first date quite like Ilana did … I appreciated that she felt comfortable enough to eat in front of me, contrary to other dates I'd experienced who picked on their lettuce and twirled their food around on the plate. I just had a feeling this was the one, and we dated for the next five years.

Getting married, living the life and starting a family

Martin and I married in 1998. He was 27 years old and I was 23. It was all going according to plan and I'd accomplished what I'd set out to do. I'd married the man of my dreams. We were both successful in our careers; made nice money; had a nice house in a nice suburb; and were ready to begin our nice family. Everything was, well … nice – and comfortable – on my road of normality.

After four years of marriage it was time to take the next step. I fell pregnant with our first child without any difficulty. My pregnancy was completely normal, and during my regular visits my gynaecologist repeatedly assured me that my baby was in perfect health.

Our firstborn's arrival

We couldn't wait for the day of David's birth. Since I was having a Caesarean, we arrived at the clinic on the date decided on by my gynaecologist – 24 June 2002. I remember standing and looking down at the empty crib in the maternity ward, waiting full of hope and excitement to see my baby finally lying there. And to take my first steps into motherhood …

I remember the Caesarean and the excitement of having a baby as if it were yesterday. On the first night I was so elated that I had a son I couldn't sleep. It was the most special moment of my life. I bonded with him instantly, played with his little fingers and experienced love as I never had before. We couldn't

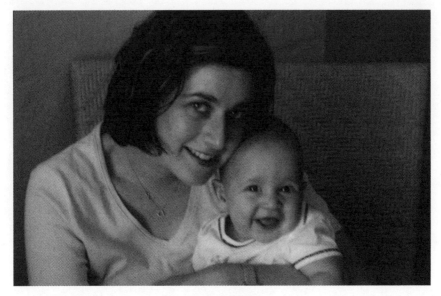

Baby David

wait to take our baby home and begin our life together as a family.

On the first night at home, all the usual cares arose: how to sterilise the bottle; whether my house was hygienic enough; how to bath and burp him. I battled with breastfeeding as David wouldn't latch.

As with any firstborn, things were a bit topsy-turvy, but I was happy, grateful and well pleased with life.

Our dream baby: June 2002–February 2004

I was the exemplary mother, taking David for his BCG, Polio, DTP, *Haemophilus influenzae* type b, Hepatitis B and MMR vaccinations on the dot at the prescribed intervals.

David was the perfect baby: he smiled, lifted his head, rolled over, sat up without support, crawled, pulled himself up into a standing position and walked at all the normal milestones. He played peek-a-boo and hide-and-seek, and loved his little blue scooter. He looked at us, and rewarded me with a huge smile when I tickled him. Apart from a little reflux at seven months, life was idyllic for the first ten months.

From ten months, he suffered from recurring ear infections that the ear, nose and throat (ENT) specialist treated with antibiotics. Pretty normal for a baby, we thought. At about 11 months, diarrhoea and a high fever that lasted for seven days landed David in hospital. The paediatrician struggled for almost two hours to find a vein in which to insert the intravenous (IV) drip ... and David fought and screamed the entire time.

We felt that this incident had really affected him adversely. When we went home, however, we suddenly noticed that our son didn't want to look at us anymore. This was frightening. He also showed no interest in playing our usual games of peek-a-boo. The laughs, smiles or reactions that 'normal' babies his age use to communicate were gone; the sparkle in his eyes had dimmed ... and the countless trips to doctors, specialists and therapists began. Life as we knew it – and as I'd so carefully planned it – was over.

No parent knows what the future has in store when they excitedly hold their newborn in their arms. For us the future would unfold like a horror story with shocks at every turn – but at the beginning we still hadn't opened the book.

Raising children presents challenges for every parent, but raising David took intense courage. In those early years, it was a one-way street of constant giving without receiving anything in return.

Therapists, specialists and increasing unease

David was 18 months old when I began my search for answers. He was unresponsive and had stopped developing. I'll never forget my first visit to an occupational therapist, one well known for her expertise with babies. David walked into her therapy room and ran around in circles. He wouldn't touch any equipment she presented him with and made no eye contact with her. She didn't speak to David and instead tried to lure him with the usual baby toys, but without success. At the end of the appointment she told me there was certainly cause for concern, briefly mentioned the word 'autism', then told me she wasn't authorised to make a diagnosis. She mentioned that most kids looked at her fleetingly at least, but that David had made no eye contact at all. She expressed the opinion that he was too young for a diagnosis and that we should come back in a few months' time.

I left the therapy room with an uneasy feeling and a heavy heart. By the time I got home, I was in tears and fear had set in.

Looking back, I wish she'd confirmed the red flags of autism right then. If we had received an official diagnosis around that time, David could have started treatment much earlier and might even have recovered. We know now that early intervention is key.

In my heart, I simply knew that David wouldn't 'grow out of it'. I'd read about the developmental milestones; and knew they were there for a reason. I felt very uneasy that David wasn't reaching them. I wasn't prepared to lose valuable time and I wasn't going to wait months to secure an appointment in search of a diagnosis. I was looking for confirmation of my worst fears, because I felt that the sooner I identified the problem, the better were my chances of improving our lives.

At that stage of our journey, though, there was always someone to reassure us – incorrectly – that he was 'a late starter and he'd soon catch up'. It couldn't be autism, right? David looked so normal …

Had we listened to this advice, it may have been another three or four years before we looked for help. We'd have lost many years of crucial intervention and development had we not taken action immediately upon discovering that David was not developing on time.

The next appointment was with the paediatrician. I described David's bowel movements and his delayed development. The paediatrician diagnosed him with toddler's diarrhoea. He assured me the frequent bowel movements were insignificant and would pass. Once again, I was dismissed without progress.

We went on to consult a speech therapist trained in neurodevelopmental treatment (NDT), whom we had been assured was the best local practitioner in the field of delayed language acquisition. David cried and screamed for most of the consultation, refused to co-operate with her and wouldn't imitate what she was doing. In a last attempt to escape the demands she placed on him, he threw himself on the floor, distressed and with his hands flapping. It crossed my mind that if she couldn't manage his behaviour, she'd likely not succeed with the therapy or its ultimate goal of speech.

David and I then flew to Bloemfontein to consult the top neurologist in South Africa. I remember sitting on the plane with David and looking through the window at the clouds, hoping I'd have answers on my journey home. Sadly, this trip didn't bring answers or the solution I'd so desperately hoped for. After seeing us for about an hour, the neurologist told me to put David onto Risperdal (a psychiatric medication) for his hyperactivity. 'Push the dose,' he said, 'you can go up to 1 mg of Risperdal.'

My gut instinct told me this wasn't the answer, and I was right. Risperdal did nothing to calm David. It just made him tired. Looking back, we realised we were giving him psychiatric medication when he was in fact a medically ill child. The neurologist mentioned in passing that we should try to get his continuous bowel movements under control. He didn't, however, make the gut–brain connection or even mention autism when the signs were so glaring.

No help anywhere

'Take him for play therapy to a psychologist specialising in children who are not social,' the voice on the other end of the phone advised. I politely agreed with my concerned friend, who was offering advice to take David for play therapy.

In our quest to do everything possible, we also took David to a psychologist who tried to engage him. He, too, was unsuccessful.

Everyone was too afraid to mention that dreaded word – 'autism'.

All the professionals from whom we sought help were unable to offer either an official diagnosis or a lasting remedy. David regressed rapidly. He'd lost his speech and the side effects of the medication caused worse problems. Behaviourally, he only made eye contact fleetingly; didn't have any imaginative or constructive play; and didn't imitate us by clapping his hands or waving. I was beside myself. We could see David's regression but could do nothing to stop it. It was like a runaway train.

After all these negative experiences, we had nothing to show. Hopelessness set in and the future seemed bleak. One relation came up with what he felt was the solution.

Put David in a home and forget about him …

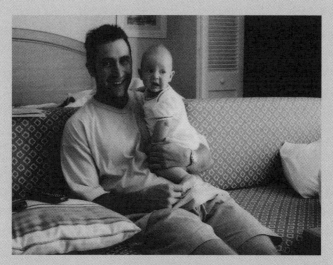

Martin and David

As David was our first child, I didn't really know what to expect. As for any new parent when you come home with a new baby, it's a bit of a minefield. When I was asked whether I was thinking about what I'd do with my son in the future, I'd answer 'not really'; I was more concerned with his immediate needs of eating and being changed. My thoughts centred around keeping a good relationship with my wife, managing my work and my child as he was back then.

When I look at that question now, I realise that I never ever experienced those dreams with David. I never had the chance to and only later did I think: 'What did I miss?' Today I can look at photos and videos of David when he was small, which were too difficult to engage with before. Now, as a father of three children and knowing so much more about what could have been, looking at them is even harder than it was originally.

I don't think we could have done more and it's simply hindsight that makes it possible to think of what could have been. This book is about hope, but there's a lot of bitterness that comes along with this story, which was and still is a very difficult journey that consumes us.

CHAPTER TWO

THE DIAGNOSIS

In February 2004, when David was about 20 months old, we visited a developmental specialist. We had to wait two agonising, soul-stealing months before we secured an appointment with her. When I close my eyes and cast my memory back to that fateful day, I can still see her sitting behind her large desk as she delivered the diagnosis that destroyed the more or less normal path we thought we were taking.

The outcome of this visit turned into a surreal nightmare from which there was no escape. What she gave us was not merely a diagnosis, it was more like a death sentence. In a perfectly calm, matter-of-fact voice, she uttered this dreadful news and advice: 'He will never speak, go to school, be toilet-trained, have friends, get married, or hold down a job. Take out an insurance policy and see a psychologist.

'I hear you're pregnant,' she added casually. 'I don't know what to tell you. I guess you can go for genetic testing. No guarantees, unfortunately.'

Her parting words to us?

'Goodbye and good luck.'

She turned and left for another appointment.

We finally had our diagnosis, delivered in cold and brutal language.

Before she spoke those fateful words, we had still had hope that everything would turn out right. Before the gavel strikes and the words leave the judge's lips, the sentence is neither legal nor official.

But now the developmental specialist's gavel had struck, the words had left her mouth, and the sentence had been pronounced.

'Autism!'

All our hope dissipated into dust.

* * *

As hope deserted us, the vacuum it left behind drew in fear and sadness ... great sadness, and a sense of loss beyond description. My idyllic dream of a happy family was shattered. At that moment, I wanted to die – with no thought of my husband, child or unborn child. I had always wanted a small gap between my kids as it would be nice for them to be close in age while growing up. It was all ruined.

As the developmental specialist dismissed us, it felt as if she'd delivered a life sentence and we left her office reeling in shock. There was no social worker, family member, parent or professional working in autism spectrum disorder (ASD) present to wipe my tears, hold my hand or offer words of wisdom; and there had certainly not been any mention of treatment options. And how did I deal with this devastating news knowing that inside me I was carrying my next child?

My beloved David had vanished into himself ... a place where I couldn't reach him.

My nice, 'normal' world collapsed. Mourning the 'death' of my firstborn, and believing I'd never be able to have a normal relationship with him, I was plunged into severe sorrow and defeat. I lay wounded on the floor, sobbing for hours on end, crying oceans of tears, mourning what felt like a living death.

The vacuum of autism

When someone you love dies, the date and time of death are recorded and everyone expects you to go through a period of mourning. You have a memory of the event and think intensely about the loved one you lost. Losing our connection with David, however, was and for a long time remained a loss that could not be quantified. There wasn't the usual support offered by our Jewish community in the event of a death – no prayer groups, meals being dropped off, or people offering encouragement. It was just Martin and I and our baby, who looked like David but wasn't David anymore.

Another reason why we experienced autism as a social vacuum was that, when we first received David's diagnosis, our initial instinct was to hide him, the label 'autism' and ourselves from the rest of the world.

Autism thus swallowed David very quickly, and it was as if it had cruelly left us with an empty shell and an unreachable soul. We still sometimes wonder when it was, exactly, that autism came to take David away from us. If we could mark a specific date, we wouldn't only remember the loss but would also have an annual 'autism is treatable' party to celebrate the victories we've experienced since then.

The period before the diagnosis was that much more unbearable because David was a first child. With a first child, you are still learning about motherhood and how to deal with a baby. You don't always know what's wrong when they become sick; and initially you panic because they can't tell you how they feel. At about three years, they may be able to tell you their tummy, ear or head hurts and life becomes easier for parents as far as being able to help their child is concerned. However, David had lost his speech – all he had left was crying and episodes of extreme behaviour. And although we didn't know it then, it would be many years before he would communicate – even his basic needs. For new parents, and particularly those who can't afford or don't receive the necessary support from professionals or family, this can be frightening, confusing and immobilising.

The typical medical problems appear

David continued to suffer from bouts of gastro. His bowel movements were explosive, frequent (eight to ten a day) and smelly, and sometimes contained mucous. For the parent this is challenging, but for the infant the physical impact is painful and uncomfortable. He'd become very hyperactive before a bowel movement. His belly was bloated and looked like an inflated balloon. This was a red flag, indicating that he was possibly suffering from yeast and bacterial overgrowth in his gut, but we had no idea then.

The ear infections also kept recurring. Of course, with the use of antibiotics, the reflux became more intense and we found ourselves regularly battling high fevers. Years later, we'd learn these medical issues were in fact a major contributor to his autism.

David also stopped developing any skills. His skin was pale, he had dark rings around his eyes and he remained sick all the time. My search to find a diagnosis and above all, solutions, now began. I involved myself in intensive research, and undertook numerous treks to specialists and therapists. The words of Nelson Mandela express what I began to realise after a while: 'I learnt that courage was not the absence of fear, but the triumph over it.'

The search for answers begins

I sprang into action as soon as we arrived home after receiving the official diagnosis that seemed to seal David's fate, and researched everything I could find on the illness that had stolen our child. I didn't know it then, but we were at the base camps of Mount Everest – with much hard work, uncertainty and treacherous terrain ahead of us before we could get close to the summit. In my determination to access treatment for David, I managed to block out all feelings of panic and started to make phone calls. A voice inside me propelled me forward, egging me on to act and preventing me from freezing. Even though I was a few weeks pregnant and nauseous, I battled the constant feeling of wanting to throw up. I sipped ginger tea to relieve the discomfort, too afraid to take anything stronger.

THE VOICE OF DOOM

My first phone call was to a South African autism organisation, whose representatives said that autism was a life-long disability. They told me to make him 'as comfortable as possible'! The only help they could suggest was a parent-support group and a brochure on autism through the post. Days later when the brochure arrived – laying out the terrible symptoms of autism, including the fact that children with autism can have seizures in their teens – I actually did throw up.

There was no mention in the brochure of any medical treatment or educational intervention. No sign of hope. No glimmer of light at the end of the tunnel. The organisation was paving a dark and gloomy road ahead for us, and I was quite astonished. I wasn't prepared to give my baby up to autism or a parent-support group. Contrary to their advice, I was not going to accept autism as a permanent disability. Looking for some lead or indication of treatment, I turned the brochure upside down but found none. There was a picture on the front of a boy with autism spinning on a merry-go-round and looking down with no eye contact; and, of course, the number of a parent-support group on the back.

This was the worst time of our lives. Instead of the happy motherhood I'd dreamt about, life became a daily travail filled with extremes of exhaustion, fear, depression and sadness. David cried and screamed constantly; he was quiet only when he slept. A heavy, ever-present grey cloud descended on me. I had no escape.

I couldn't eat or sleep, buy new clothes or even look at myself in the mirror. I used no make-up and barely felt alive. Friends suggested I seek professional help for myself, but I wasn't emotionally ready for this. I first had to mourn the loss of David's normal development and kept all my emotions safely locked away. It took time before I could talk about my shattered dreams, fear and brokenness.

The journey to the return of hope began when we started to educate ourselves about autism. We read everything we could find: what autism is; what causes it; and, most of all, how to not only stop but also *turn around* the regression we'd witnessed in David.

A first ray of hope

In our search for answers, one of the first books we read was *Children with Starving Brains: A Medical Treatment Guide for Autism Spectrum Disorder*, written by the late Dr Jaquelyn McCandless. Both Martin and I read her book multiple times and became very excited on recognising many of David's problems. We tracked down Dr McCandless in the United States, phoned her and asked for a consultation. Her response was that she was now semi-retired and was not taking on any new patients. We sent her a photo of our beautiful baby with his big eyes and blonde curls, along with some South African curios, in an attempt to make an impression and convince her to change her mind. It worked and she finally agreed to consult with us.

BIOMEDICAL TESTING

For a start, Dr McCandless told us, we would need to provide her with David's urine, blood, stool and hair for analysis. She sent us the testing kits, which came accompanied by detailed use instructions from the US laboratories. Martin studied the collection guides carefully, and we prepared ourselves for the daunting task of drawing blood and meeting the stringent requirements set out in the kits' guidelines. We arranged for our paediatrician to draw the blood because we wanted to make sure we left no room for error. On the morning of the appointment, he was called away to an emergency and his partner, a well-recognised paediatrician, stood in for him.

I remember sitting at the clinic as we waited 45 minutes for him to arrive. David was crying for his bottle, which I couldn't give him because we had to wait for the blood to be drawn before he could break his fast. For a normal child this is difficult – for David it was unthinkable. When the paediatrician arrived and prepared his equipment, he snapped at me angrily, saying he'd agreed to stand in for his partner but wanted me to know he was against the tests. This even though he had received no proper training on the subject at medical school!

Afterwards, as David cried and screamed, Martin rushed the blood specimen to a laboratory so it could be centrifuged into the components required by the laboratories in the United States.

Not only was Martin carrying a precious cargo – it was also not a normal sample drop-off. We had to make sure that our local lab understood the samples' significance and the care that needed to go into preparing them. We knew there was no way we could put David through the same thing again soon. There was no room for error.

I took David home while Martin went to a specialised courier service to package and label the samples. Some of these had to be frozen, others had to be refrigerated and yet others were to be kept at room temperature. Martin filled out reams of paperwork requiring him to describe the samples and the reasons for the testing. I nervously waited for his call. Finally, he let me know it had all worked out and we'd been successful in getting the samples off.

When he arrived home, however, we realised that the laboratory had performed the blood centrifuge at the wrong speed. My heart sank. Later that evening, we called the US laboratory to report this. Thankfully, they said they'd accept the blood despite the incorrect speed.

One of the blood samples had to arrive at a laboratory in Beverly Hills within 24 hours of being drawn. We held out little hope this would happen, but fortunately it arrived on time and we breathed a sigh of relief.

All we could do now was to wait for the test results.

* * *

When Dr McCandless's report arrived, it was a relief to see that it went into satisfying detail, and not just about what was wrong with David:

> *The results show marked gastric pathology. His gut is deeply infiltrated with pathogenic bacteria and yeast that need intensive treatment. This includes natural and prescriptive medications as indicated. He needs to have any offending foods that could encourage gut inflammation removed, including wheat, milk and refined sugar.*
>
> *David has heavy metals poisoning and needs corrective minerals. Glutathione IVs would benefit him greatly. His gut is currently not absorbing vital nutrients. After gut health is on its way, chelation should be considered.*
>
> *David's testing reveals gross deficiencies in many of his primary nutrients, especially amino acids, B-vitamins and other anti-oxidants.*
>
> *Current viral infection in the form of high herpes antibodies, with evidence of autoimmunity per positive brain autoantibodies, has been detected.*

At the end of her report she had added: '*This completes my evaluation of your son; there are many things you can do to help your son start to get much, much better. I wish you the very best in the healing of your precious little boy.*

Jaquelyn McCandless, M.D.'

That night, I couldn't sleep. Her words kept going around and around in my head – 'I wish you the very best in the *healing* of your precious little boy.' It was the first time since our journey with autism had begun that anyone had offered us a glimmer of hope.

We had finally found the answers we were looking for; we could start fighting back, and embark on our journey of starting to treat David's medical problems.

Before this report, the 'devil' had had no face – now we could clearly see what we were fighting against. Nothing was going to stop us winning this war.

At last, we were no longer enveloped in grey – light was there, albeit still at the end of a long tunnel.

CHAPTER THREE

DISCOVERING APPLIED BEHAVIOURAL ANALYSIS

Even though we had made progress, every day was still as painful as ever. David presented with all the symptoms labelled 'autism' that I'd been reading about. How I dreaded that word! I'd watch as he'd line up his toys in a long row, and flap his hands while watching *Barney* over and over again on our television set. I soon realised that these behaviours amounted to the Autism 101 textbook. If we had any visitors at the house, he'd line them up in a row, forcing our guests to remain sitting in the order in which he'd organised them. If anyone dared to get up, he'd fetch them and place them back in line. We stopped inviting people over to our house for fear of having to deal with David's behaviour.

Applied Behavioural Analysis (ABA)

Having done my training at a prestigious law firm, I was well versed in research techniques. I turned on my laptop and the hunt for solutions began.

I found a South African organisation that specialised in ABA and supplied a number to call. I spoke to them for about 20 minutes and felt relieved by our conversation. ABA made sense to me instantly. They said they would be presenting a course on ABA the following week in Johannesburg and invited me to attend, after which they would start David on an ABA programme. David was only 20 months old and they explained that early intervention was important. The call reassured me that not all hope was lost and I felt soothed by the exchange and promise of help.

Three weeks later, at the tender age of 21 months, David embarked on his ABA journey. A team of three girls trained in ABA methodology arrived at my house to set up his programme. I received a long list of items we'd need and prepared his ABA room. I bought him a purple wooden table and chairs, and arranged all his toys in order. Up to this point everything we had asked of David or tried to get him to do had been on his terms. He wasn't pointing, which is a prerequisite to language acquisition, and his ability to imitate others' behaviours was non-existent. He wasn't making the normal baby talk sounds (such as b and c for ball and car). I had been asked to collect items that were highly motivating for David; and had bought every single *Barney* video in the shop in preparation for ABA.

David was non-compliant and at the same time hyperactive. He walked into his new ABA room and made no eye contact with his ABA team. Instead, he started spinning in circles. The three girls assigned to David – Candy, Jacqui and Janine – tried to engage with him on the floor. Candy took David by the hand and sat him down opposite her on the chair, holding her legs around his to prevent him running away. She placed a tray on her lap so they had a hard surface to work on. His first target was to imitate placing a block in a bucket.

They explained that their first step would be to teach David to imitate; and that we'd move on to more complicated imitation targets such as gross and fine motor imitation once David had mastered a sufficient number of object imitations. We'd build to vocal imitation, but before we got there we had to make sure that other developmental milestones were in place.

Candy gave David a yellow bucket and a red block. She turned his face to hers, waited for him to make some eye contact, and followed this up with the standard instruction for imitative behaviour: 'Do this.' She then performed the action – which David was supposed to imitate – of placing the block in the bucket.

David was given one second in which to respond. He didn't, and so Candy prompted him to imitate what she'd just done by placing her hand on his while she guided him in placing the block in the bucket. David

wasn't co-operating and became hysterical, arching his back and screaming loudly.

David found a weapon to fight back with. He cried so much he threw
up all over Candy and himself. A first reaction normally might be to pay
attention to this behaviour, but I was prepped to ignore it and we cleaned
him and the room up without uttering a word or showing the least reaction. This felt unnatural and painful. My baby had just thrown up all over
himself and the floor, and I had to behave as if nothing had happened. I
could feel the team's eyes on me; and I had to control my reactions and true
feelings and go along with the plan. This wasn't easy.

David didn't only throw up once. He vomited another 10 times, and I
gathered a heap of clothes in the corner of the room to be able to change
his clothes each time. Every time he threw up we'd get up, clean up, change
him and sit him back down again. It was one of the worst days of my life.

My next-door neighbour heard the continuous crying and screaming.
As I'd forgotten to confide in her that David had autism and that I was
starting an ABA programme, she thought we were under attack and that
something bad was happening to my family. She phoned me a few times but
I didn't answer. Then she knocked on the door and I didn't open. Finally,
she dialled my mobile and I had to pick up. I was cleaning the vomit with
one hand and speaking to her on the phone with the other.

When I finally answered she asked, 'Ilana is everything okay? I hear
David crying and screaming – what's going on – have you been tied up
and robbed?' I didn't know what to say. I was rushed, and so told her very
quickly that we were okay and that I'd explain everything later. She told me
she had been considering calling the police, and was glad I'd finally picked
up the call.

When I put down the phone, I felt embarrassed. To make matters worse,
her daughter had been born the day before David and I had witnessed her
develop and acquire speech effortlessly. I'll never forget the day when, at 18
months, she called my name, pronouncing it perfectly. I remember secretly
and desperately wishing that David could do that too.

Odious comparison
'Comparison is the thief of joy.' – *Theodore Roosevelt*

That night, when everyone had gone home and I could enjoy the tranquil peace of darkness and silence, I collapsed crying on the couch. I sobbed and sobbed for a very long time. I was hunched over in a foetal position with my head buried under the cushion as my body shook from the uncontrollable sorrow I felt. I wished my life could end. The only thing to which I could equate what I'd experienced was taming a wild horse. No parent should have to witness what I went through that day and this was only the beginning. My little baby with his soft peach skin, whom we had brought home from the hospital with his ten toes and ten fingers, who had lain sleeping like an angel in white lace in a carry cot in my bedroom, was lost to me. The smell of baby, the softness of his baby blankets and our perfect world with him had been ripped from us so early on … I still struggle to look at his baby pictures; and when I do, I am overcome by feelings of deep sadness and pain.

A tough regime
David would start ABA at 7 am sharp every day from Monday to Friday. When we took a break before the afternoon session (which stretched from 2.30 till 4.30 pm), I'd rock him to sleep in a hammock and place him wrapped in it on my bed. Being pregnant made me feel tired and, although I didn't dare sleep during the day, I'd lie down on the floor in my dark walk-in cupboard to escape from the world. I felt safe on the hard floor in the darkness, where I could block out the world for a few minutes. I used every free waking moment I had to read books on autism and research treatments for it. David's diet and medical protocol required my constant attention and there was by no means enough time to sleep.

For seven hours of each day for the first three months of the ABA treatment, I didn't leave David's side. I remained in his ABA room with him and with his team, who took turns working with him. I couldn't pull myself away, not even for one minute, holding my breath as we worked through his lessons. I sat on the floor and watched them closely. David eventually started to imitate actions with objects; and we soon moved on to gross motor imitation such as waving and clapping one's hands.

I'll never forget trying to get David to clap his hands. We had brainstormed this behavioural target inside out. I turned on his favourite *Barney* movie, pausing it at his favourite part. David looked angrily at Candy and me. She delivered the command, 'Do this,' then clapped her hands. What happened next was unbelievable: David proceeded to clap his hands. We turned the movie back on within a second of his executing the instruction, and found ourselves screaming with joy. That had been a real victory, and we did a celebratory dance around the room. I started to get the hang of ABA, realising that if the reward was big enough, David would try his very best to follow the instruction.

More than a glimmer of hope

David was making progress. Initially, we'd hold all the objects to which he wanted access to our faces, in order to get him to make eye contact with us. Once his eyes met mine, I'd release the desired item. David loved his dummy and we sometimes used it as a reward. When I passed him his dummy or water bottle, I'd make sure to hold these objects to my face to prompt him to look at my eyes. If we called his name and he didn't respond, we'd physically turn his face to ours for a response. Over time David started to respond to his name.

Jacqui, Candy and Janine treated every session very seriously. They'd take turns working with David, alternating daily. If Candy took the morning session, Janine took the one in the afternoon. I would rush to get him ready for these afternoon sessions. Candy was stern and David knew he'd be expected to work hard during her scheduled session times. They had a certain mutual respect and understanding, and I knew David trusted her. Janine was lots of fun, and David seemed to really enjoy spending time with her. But he loved Jacqui most of all. Firstly, she was blonde, and David liked blonde girls. And while she was no push-over, she spoke gently to him, and he'd do things for her he wouldn't do for me or the rest of the team.

After four months on the programme, we took stock. David had learnt to make eye contact, started to respond to his name, no longer did everything only on his terms and had mastered the imitation that was a prerequisite to vocal imitation. We were stuck on a lesson called object discrimination, which is often hard for children with autism to grasp. In order to get David to speak, we had to teach him to form physical sounds and words, putting together consonants and vowels. We also needed to teach him a vocabulary of words he could use to communicate.

Other challenges

TREATING DAVID'S ABNORMAL SLEEP PATTERNS

Seeking to improve David's very poor sleep patterns over the years included treating many problems common to children with autism, including:

- ❏ Gastrointestinal issues and acid reflux
- ❏ Vitamin and/or mineral deficiencies (especially the mineral magnesium)
- ❏ Below-average levels of melatonin
- ❏ Automatic nervous system dysfunction
- ❏ High levels of yeast and/or parasites

HAVING TO BE WITH DAVID ALL THE TIME

You could never just leave David on his own. Added to the physical hardships was the problem of keeping him permanently occupied. A normal child can take a spoon and turn it into a car and have fun. Even with an abundance of toys around him, though, David wasn't interested in anything other than sitting in a corner and being destructive. He just broke everything within his reach. If you gave him a toy, he'd find a way to rip it apart. If you left him alone on the couch, he'd unpick a seam ...

We had to find a way to supervise David every single second of every day. That was a hardship then and still is today. David can't be left alone, which means that someone has to be with him all the time.

Intensifying ABA

Although David made significant gains, he was stuck in the area of vocal imitation. If he struggled to master a target, we'd try many different ways to get him to grasp the concept. We were trying to teach David that the word 'shoe' referred to a shoe and that the word 'cup' was assigned to a cup, but he wasn't making a connection between the spoken word and the object. When we placed both a shoe and a cup in front of him and asked him to pass the shoe to Candy, it was challenging for him.

This lesson became very frustrating for David. When I walked down the passage leading to his ABA room, I could hear Candy working on object discrimination. 'Give me shoe, give me cup,' her voice rotated through the different targets. I'd often sit outside the door, my back to the wall and a prayer book in my hand, begging for mercy and results.

A BAD IDEA

I started working with David too and became quite successful at getting him to master his ABA targets. I knew him best and no one cared more for him than me. It made sense to familiarise myself with the principles of ABA and I became part of his team of therapists.

This was a bad idea and I would later come to regret my decision. There was too much at stake. I had so much vested in him being successful – and my emotions clouded my intellect. I had to be his mom, not his therapist, and ABA ruined our relationship. I pushed him too far and couldn't be objective. I only made the situation worse, as shown by the fact that David became afraid to select an answer. To be one of his primary therapists, undertaking the role of a teacher, wasn't viable.

After a few years I took what felt like a decision to step down as his therapist. While it was difficult for me to delegate his progress and future to his team, I had come to realise that it was important.

Eli's birth, September 2004

I have no idea how we survived the nine months of pregnancy, living as we were with so much uncertainty and no guarantee that Eli would be autism-free.

NOT YOUR AVERAGE PREGNANCY

During the early days of ABA, I was dealing not only with David's trauma but also with the extra hormones of my pregnancy with Eli. It wasn't unusual for Martin to arrive home and find me crying. He knew why I was crying and didn't need to ask for a reason. If he didn't find me crying, it had been a particularly good day, with some new lead or article on the treatment of autism lifting my spirits and drying my tears. I was very cautious during my pregnancy with Eli not to swallow anything harmful. I developed severe toothache and needed root-canal treatment to save my tooth. To the dismay of my dentist, I refused an anaesthetic and he fixed my tooth while I squeezed the armrests of the chair to deal with the pain and noise of his drill. I didn't take a single painkiller during my pregnancy.

David, now two years and three months, had been delivered by Caesarean section and I was therefore not going to attempt a natural birth. I had a few days to go before my second booked Caesarean. My feet were swollen as I sat on the floor in David's ABA room going over his data and lessons with a fine toothcomb.

AN EMOTIONAL BIRTH

On the morning we checked into the Park Lane Clinic, Martin and I took the lift to the maternity ward in silence. There were no words to describe our emotions. I remember seeing Eli's tiny face in an incubator just after he arrived. There was a long scratch down the side of his face from the forceps the paediatrician had used to pull him out. He looked completely different from David, as he had dark skin and a chiselled face.

The paediatrician was performing the Apgar test in the corner of the recovery room. On hearing him speak to the nurses, I immediately became concerned that something was wrong. At that moment he walked over to us, and said he was putting Eli in the incubator with a device to assist his breathing as there was some water on his lungs. He told us that if the breathing didn't normalise in a few minutes he'd admit him to the neonatal intensive-care unit. After a tense couple of minutes, however, Eli's breathing normalised. He achieved an Apgar score of 10/10, and was released into my care.

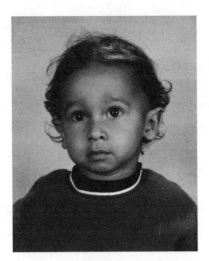

Baby Eli

I held Eli in the recovery room before being wheeled back to the ward. He latched onto my breast immediately, knowing instinctively what to do. Breastfeeding him wasn't at all challenging. This was very different from my experience with David, who didn't latch and struggled to feed. In that moment when Eli latched effortlessly, I knew he'd be okay. Spending two nights in hospital felt like spending time in a hotel. The nurses brought me cups of tea and snacks, and checked on my every need. I hadn't been away from David since he had been born and I enjoyed the break away.

COMING HOME

I brought my newborn son to a house where a home-based ABA programme saw therapists coming in and out every waking moment of the day. David screamed most days and Eli had to learn to sleep through the noise. Our fast day of Yom Kippur, one of the most important days in the Jewish calendar, was slowly approaching. Although Jewish law didn't require me to fast strictly for 24 hours with no food or water as I'd just delivered a baby, I decided to fast anyway. Eli was four days old and I stood in his room for most of the day reciting the traditional prayers. Later that evening, I broke my fast with Martin at the scheduled time. Always aware I had to continue to work on my spiritual growth, I hoped my efforts would secure health and well-being for my family. I didn't struggle to fast, as on most days I didn't eat much anyway. Worrying about David filled my mind, body and soul – there was no room for food.

Eli was one week old and David needed to get out of the house. My doctor had given me strict instructions not to drive for at least six weeks after the Caesarean. However, I had no time to recuperate or think about not driving and taking it easy. I climbed into the car with David and took him to the park. I didn't think about the physical pain or possible consequences of driving so soon after the Caesar.

A bad scare with our new baby

At four months of age Eli contracted a debilitating rotavirus that made him throw up multiple times. I rushed him to the paediatrician. Not wanting to take any chances with a small baby, he inserted an infusion needle into Eli's arm to keep him hydrated and admitted him to hospital. I sat in the chair next to my son for five days and five nights, until we were discharged and sent home. Back home David was also unwell, not from a rotavirus but from his chronic bowl disease and diarrhoea. When Martin relieved me for a few hours so I could go home and check on David, I found my son pale and withdrawn, curled on the bed in his room. My heart broke to see David this way and we had to muster all our strength and faith to get through these tough periods.

Trying out playschool for David

We spent a year on the South African ABA programme. We gave it our best shot, and David made definite intellectual gains. However, he remained sick most of the time despite the fact that we were juggling various medical treatments. As a result, we decided to take a break from ABA and to focus on David's health and an effective medical protocol. But it was a mistake to stop ABA. The two treatments go hand in hand, and this was another decision we would come to regret. Looking back, this was one of the worst choices we ever made.

We also decided it was time for David to experience school; and made an appointment to meet the headmistress of a local playschool. The place was everything we could have dreamt of or hoped for when choosing a school, and the teacher he was to be allocated to was clearly passionate about teaching children. We told the head that David had autism and asked that he be allowed in with a facilitator present. Her initial reaction was to give us all the reasons why her school wouldn't be the right placement for him. Martin insisted that we wanted David to be considered just like any other child might be. Reluctantly, she found it in her heart to give David a chance and accepted him on a trial basis. Candice Breetzke, one of his ABA team members, agreed to be his facilitator, and David spent a year in playschool. Initially, David thrived in the playschool's warm and loving environment and under Candice's protective wing. But as the months went by, the cracks in his development became more prominent and we grew steadily more uneasy. The gaps between David and his peers were becoming wider and wider. In our hearts we came to realise that, as much as the playschool had agreed to accommodate us, David needed more. As the year came to a close and I walked away from the school on the last day, I knew we were in trouble.

The ABA team's views on its intervention in David's case

CANDICE BREETZKE, BOARD CERTIFIED AUTISM TECHNICIAN
Before I relate my experience of implementing ABA with David, I have to stress that therapy in any form can only be successful if parents are dedicated to implementing strategies at home, outside of therapy. David is blessed with wonderfully dedicated and passionate parents.

I was greeted at 7 in the morning by the most beautiful, curly-haired, two-year-old boy. My heart melted, and I was in love and totally ready to teach this little gem to learn. Despite his qualities, however, David was no easy boy to teach. He put up a battle that surely gave his parents their money's worth. He wouldn't sit, and succeeded in biting and badly bruising me. He also got sick all over me – all in an attempt to resist the unwelcome onslaught of behaviour modification. I can only imagine that his parents, Martin and Ilana, found this both incredibly trying and heartbreaking. But their persistence and dedication never waned.

Fortunately, with perseverance and by choosing the most effective rewards, we were able to get little David to sit and make eye contact within a period of three days. David made remarkable progress. He would do anything for a jump on the trampoline.

His ability to imitate when rewarded appropriately was fantastic, and he quickly learnt to clap, wave and so forth. He began to recognise and match first one, then two, then three pictures at a time. His receptive language and ability to follow simple one-step instructions blossomed. Within a short period of time, we were able to move from tangible food rewards to rewarding him with short clips from *Barney* DVDs (to this day I know every *Barney* song there is).

David soon progressed to enjoying verbal praise and high fives. We were also able to change from having the door permanently closed (so David couldn't escape) to working with an open door. We moved on from working only at the table to having more fun and different learning opportunities on the floor. David's expressive language was a little slower to develop, but he slowly started to approximate sounds in order to gain access to activities that he wanted to do – so that the activity itself became the reward.

As part of the programme, David was also put on a strict diet and I noticed a positive change. He was so blessed to have a mom who meticulously monitored his diet and provided him with the correct, healthy food. David's parents explored a biomedical approach and this too had many benefits.

It's obvious that in order to maximise a child's potential, intervention needs to be multifaceted. Another important component is the large number of hours involved, as the more input a child receives from as early as possible, the greater the progress and long-term benefits.

Working with David and his parents was truly a privilege and a very rewarding experience.

JANINE CLARK, BOARD CERTIFIED AUTISM TECHNICIAN
I remember the first day I met Ilana and David. It was a hot summer's afternoon in Johannesburg. I vividly remember jumping on the trampoline with David in the garden at Martin and Ilana's home.

My dear friend Jacqui had introduced me to Ilana and David. As a young undergraduate psychology student, I was very excited to have the opportunity to be exposed to some practical work. Little did I know then that my life and education would take on a new direction. I arrived with some very stereotyped ideas of what autism was and how it was treated, but little David with his gentle soul captivated me and taught me more than any university course could ever teach me.

I was blessed to be able to join the ABA team who worked with David in those early days of his journey. I've always seen David's journey as a mountain-range hike that I joined in one of the first valleys.

I have a few vivid memories from those early days of therapy with David. His sessions took place in his home, where a therapy room had been created in one of the bedrooms.

Sessions started at 7 am and ran through to around 5 pm with a nap-time break for David. So the days were intense for him as well as his parents. I always thought that running the therapy in their home was both a blessing and a curse for Ilana.

I remember opening the door of the therapy room one day after a particularly loud tantrum of David's. There was Ilana sitting on the passage floor, pregnant with Eli, just waiting for the session to be over. I can only imagine the anguish and conflict she must have experienced. As a mother, your instinct is to run to comfort your child when they cry; and here she was being asked day in and day out to step back and not comfort her baby.

Progress was slow – we spent weeks teaching David to discriminate between objects and object labels. The two labels that have stuck with me to this day are 'book' and 'shoe'. We did trial after trial of 'touch book, no, touch book ...' and 'touch shoe, no, touch shoe ...'. In some sessions he got it right, in other sessions he just couldn't, and not because he wasn't trying; he always tried so hard. We also worked on echoics [the vocal imitation discussed earlier] and the sound we spent hours working on was 'b'. We tried everything from swinging; to bouncing; to jumping; to putting bubbles on his lips to draw sounds out. Again, David always tried, but as the sessions went on it became clear to me that while he had been diagnosed as autistic, there was something else at play. He was physically ill.

One afternoon he started to cry and, as we'd been trained, we worked through the behaviour. Then at one point something said to me that this cry was different: this was a cry of pain, not one of 'this is hard for me'. We called Ilana and she came home and immediately took David to the doctor.

This is one of the biggest challenges with autistic children – knowing the difference between them being really ill and simply wanting to escape a task. This is why you truly need an expert ABA team who are properly trained to distinguish between these different scenarios. Bad ABA can do so much damage.

David was the first child on the autism spectrum who I had the privilege to work with; and my experience with him always reminds me to see the child and not just the condition.

Martin and Ilana's dedication to finding the right treatment for David is on another level. If moving mountains could help David and others with autism, mountains would be moved. I continue to be moved by their dedication to [the care of people with] autism.

JACQUI VAN VUUREN

If I reflect now on my experiences with David, the first word that pops into my mind is 'peaceful'. [My working on the team] wasn't about a job that needed to be done, but about two individuals with their own personalities sitting opposite each other working together in our world and quietly celebrating each little achievement. As small as he was, David was smart! And learnt very quickly that the correct behaviour would elicit a favourable response that was rewarding for both of us. (Except when the reward was *Barney*. That was just for him …)

I remember knowing instinctively when David liked something and when he didn't. The speech therapist and her rooms weren't a favourite thing with him. However, being on the swing outside in the garden during a break, with the lovely winter sun on our backs, was a small pleasure even if it made going back into the therapy room a little harder.

All in all, I have such positive memories of my experiences with David and the feeling of love was so evident in the Gerschlowitz home that I'd often sit with my own children when they were that age and emulate what I would have done in the therapy room with David.

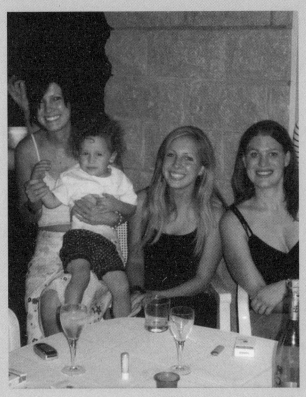

David and his team

A different take on things: Martin's story continued

HELL ON EARTH

Watching David during those early days of ABA was unbearable. It was an unnatural, horrible time in our lives. To see your child go through that is very painful and changed us as people. We couldn't expect to be the same again and it changed our relationship with David. For me this was when David's and my relationship began to change, even though he was so young.

It was harder for Ilana, because even though she was his mother she'd become his therapist and teacher, demanding so much from him both in the 'classroom' and out. She wanted him to be able to fit in with us and not the other way around. Sadly, I think it strained Ilana's relationship with him. She became 95 per cent teacher and 5 per cent mother. Her main focus was that if she could fix him, make him right, then that was the ultimate love she could show him. If he could function normally in society then he would have a future, some kind of a life.

LOVE WASN'T ENOUGH

For me it was exactly the opposite. I just thought that I needed to love my child. He was still my boy. He was still cute. He looked normal and his gross motor skills were good: he could still climb, jump on a trampoline and ride a bike. We did fun things together.

For Ilana I know finding that initial ABA was a huge breakthrough but I see it differently. It was one big slog, with David screaming and screaming through each session for hours on end. For every hour of ABA, he would scream for 50 minutes. I don't know how Ilana stood it as she sat either with him or listening at the door. I couldn't take it. As parents we believed this was a means to an end, but what did we, as first-time parents, really know when we were told that 'This is ABA and it works'? 'This is the method that will benefit your child.'

When we looked at the theory, the literature and the information we were given, it made sense. But ABA shouldn't have a child crying for hours and hours. That was a mistake. Yes, there may be moments of screaming and shouting to get over certain battles, which is normal, but for the most part the child should be happy, motivated and want to be there. David didn't want to be there. He hated every second.

SMALL STEPS

At the time I just tried to love David for who he was. I had to fit in with the code and be as consistent as I could, even though I was losing my child. He just wasn't there. You couldn't even teach him to put a block in a bucket or clap his hands. It took four months of blood, sweat, a lot of vomit and tears just to get him to clap. The most basic things, ones that people take for granted, we made a celebration of. For us it was one small thing on a long, long journey.

ABA highlights all the skills David doesn't have, so you really mourn and are very sad because you realise how much you've lost and how little he can do compared to other kids. It's very hard for a parent to go through this, when you see so many deficits and you're meant to carry on functioning – going to work, making a living.

Added to everything else, Ilana was pregnant with Eli, and the situation was so far removed from most women's second pregnancy! Most pregnant women get tired, but for Ilana the ABA intervention took exhaustion to a whole new level. Without help she literally couldn't get off her bed unaided she was so drained. She also hardly ate. She was literally deficient in calories.

TREADING ON GLASS

For most people, expecting a child comes with expectation and excitement. For us that time around, what we felt was anxiety and we didn't enjoy it for one single second. Even after our second son was born we were so engrossed with David we didn't have time to think about Eli and what was going on in his life or what he needed. Eli had to fit in with our circumstances, and before we looked around his childhood had come and gone.

Not to say we weren't worried about him. Firstly, we had decided not to vaccinate him and so had to be careful where we took him. One day he broke out in red spots all over his body and we were overcome by the fear that he'd contracted measles. We rushed him off to the doctor, who reassured us that it was only a viral rash. This incident was very stressful to deal with on top of everything else we were going through. We thought carefully about what he ate; what water and milk to give him.

We were panicked with Eli. When he got sick the question was – do we give him antibiotics or not? When he had a fever, we worried this would bring on autism. We were constantly in fear of anything triggering autism, as had happened with David.

Only when Eli was around four years old could I see his development was much better and more advanced than David's. Still the worry didn't leave us. During school plays I'd look at him to see if he was clapping as much as the other kids. Was he performing as well as the rest of the kids? I was scrutinising his every move and my standards were high. Bringing up Eli and having to deal with David at the same time was very difficult.

A COPING MECHANISM FOR ILANA

Apart from when she was pregnant, one of the ways Ilana coped was by smoking – copiously … This normally would have been really hard for me to accept as I'm a fitness and health fanatic. I find smoking disgusting; and the smell on someone else really horrible. Under any other circumstance I would have put my foot down, but I knew it helped get her through every day. Rather smoking than taking medication or hardcore drugs to get through.

After smoking for years, she finally realised it was doing more harm than good, and at that stage she didn't need it as much and stopped.

HINDSIGHT

Looking back, would we do the original local ABA again? Part of me wants to say that everything happens for a reason and there must have been a reason why we did it. It led us to a certain path and gave us hope at that time – and to be fair, David was a very, very hard case. So can I say this ABA was bad? No, but it was bad for David, whereas another child may have flourished on that programme and done well. David was a tough nut.

Even on the later CARD ABA, although he didn't scream and shout, he was extremely difficult – way more than any other child on the programme.

David was extremely defiant, opposing and rejecting everything we tried to teach him. He just wanted to be left alone to sit in a corner and do nothing the entire day. That would have made him happy. If you interrupted him when he was in his corner – that was massive. He just wanted to be. I don't think I've ever seen any other children quite like David.

THE AGONY OF EATING

For a parent to watch their child literally waste away from lack of food is unthinkable. Who would do that? Never mind that you want your child to have the most nutritious and sensible food, but to see them not eat at all is heartbreaking. Each mealtime, trying to get David to eat anything was agonising. He refused to eat, turning his face away and becoming hysterical when presented with a plate of food. His refusal was non-negotiable.

First there was the preparation: just finding gluten-, casein-, soya- and sugar-free foods was a mission in itself, apart from the preparation and cooking of the meals. Then you put it in front of him and he didn't want to eat. So if you didn't want him to waste away, you had to force him to eat or even put him on a feeding tube.

Eventually, exhausted, we thought we wouldn't force him and would let him tell us when he was hungry. He went for two to three days without anything crossing his lips except water; and at that point we realised we had to do it our way, otherwise he'd starve to death.

Then this beautiful food you'd prepared and shoved down him would most of the time be vomited up and you were back to square one. It would take around an hour to feed him, bite by bite by bite. Then he'd throw up and we'd have to bathe and change him, prepare another meal and go through the whole thing again.

We're talking three or four meals a day, seven days a week, 365 days a year. Once Eli was born, to add to the chaos, we also had bottles to prepare and nappies to change. Your child needs to eat – it's the most basic instinct but it took everything we had just to feed David.

SLEEPING

Everyone knows that one of the most important elements of a child's growth is a good night's sleep. In David's case, this was doubly important as every morning he faced his crucial ABA sessions. If he was even a little bit rattier, instead of screaming for 50 minutes he'd scream for 55 minutes and the session would be a total waste. It was crucial he slept.

And it wasn't just David who needed sleep, but the whole family. When we didn't get any sleep, how were we expected to function, work and remain sane? This tore us apart. I was a zombie.

I remembered an incident from when I was a teenager, hearing of a friend's father who had fallen asleep behind the wheel of his car. Back then I thought: 'How irresponsible! Who would do that?' I would know soon enough. There were a number of times when, sleep-deprived, I'd be driving and would have to stop at the side of the road, have a coffee or just close my eyes for a while. Ilana and I were both totally sleep-deprived and utterly exhausted. The miracle is that we didn't tear each other apart, given the lack of patience we must have experienced. Somehow, we got through the 'zombified' state we were living in. We barely existed. It was a very challenging time.

Normally with small children, parents get time together when the kids have gone to bed. For us this didn't exist. There was no 'down time' during which we could talk to each other and be a little human. David wouldn't go to sleep and was up at all hours of the night. It was soul-destroying. We couldn't even have that little bit of peace at the end of a day. Eventually, when we managed to get his medical condition under control, he'd go to bed at 9 pm or 10 pm at night, and suddenly we had this magic tranquillity, even if just for a few hours. Sometimes this was short-lived, with David waking again just after we fell asleep – and it wasn't as though we could just leave him unattended in his room …

CHAPTER FOUR

AUTISM IS TREATABLE

Like most people whose children receive a diagnosis of autism, we had been led to believe that David's autism was a lifelong neurological condition we just had to accept. But as a result of all the evidence-based research I'd done, we had begun to discover that there was a link between his autistic symptoms and his medical challenges. We now finally had direction and could start the treatments we'd read about in Dr McCandless's book.

Determined to improve David's quality of life and ours, we embarked on a brave journey along a difficult road of medical treatments. Yet I felt as if we'd applied to court to appeal the verdict of a lifelong sentence – and had won the appeal!

Brains on fire

Delving into the research, I discovered that children with autism often suffer from brain inflammation. Investigating what triggered David's inflammation in the brain was pivotal in deciding on an appropriate course of treatment. For David, this was the first step in healing his broken brain.

To hear your child has neuro-inflammation (inflammation of the nervous tissue) is difficult to come to terms with. However, things start to make sense once you start understanding why it may be present.

One of the things I discovered is that autism is 'epigenetic', i.e. 'relating to or arising from non-genetic influences on gene expression'. Stated more accessibly, it means that a genetic predisposition coupled with environmental triggers may lead to autism.

These triggers may include:
- ❏ Infections
- ❏ Environmental factors in food, air and water
- ❏ Seasonal changes (e.g. pollen)
- ❏ Toxins, ranging from air pollution to medications, and so on

Children with autism: the yellow canaries of our planet

Children with autism have been labelled our planet's 'canaries in the coal mine'. Just as canaries taken into coal mines by miners in previous years warned them of the presence of dangerous gases such as carbon monoxide and methane (they were more sensitive to the gases than the miners and got ill first), children with autism are sounding a warning for the rest of us. Their very important message is that our world is simply too toxic for healthy living, and that this toxicity is increasing both local and global prevalence of the condition.

Children with autism are more sensitive and the first to be affected by the ever-increasing toxicity of our planet. According to Professor Martha Herbert:[1]

> To say that people with autism are 'canaries in the coal mine' is to say that the problems faced by people with autism are part of a class of problems that will affect more and more people if present trends of pollution and chronic disease continue. Autism thus becomes a wake-up call.
>
> This point of view is based on the belief that at least a substantial proportion of the increase in reported cases of autism represents a true increase, and on the belief that environmental factors are contributing to this increase.

I now had renewed hope and a spring in my step. We planned our attack on autism carefully and meticulously. Finding a medical doctor who would truly listen to us and who was open to learning about the treatments was a

---

1 Source: http://www.autismwhyandhow.org/what-is-autism/canary-in-coal-mine/, accessed 11 April 2019

real breakthrough. I knew we'd need the assistance of a local doctor. I was referred to the late Dr Rodney Unterslak who, I was told, would be just the right doctor for us.

Dr Rodney instantly agreed to help us. He also jumped at the opportunity of travelling overseas, meeting Dr McCandless and shadowing her, learning about the medical complexities and treatments of autism. On his return to South Africa, he carried us through a very difficult time.

He called me at 7 am and 7 pm daily for over a year without fail, checking on David's health and progress. He was an incredible doctor and healer. We were privileged to have him on our side, supporting us. We were in a battle with autism, determined to win. Whenever we stumbled, he'd pick us up. Dr Rodney always reminded me that faith and hope would find a way. His words of wisdom taught me an important principle: 'G-d created the cure before the disease,' he would say. 'G-d has already provided the remedy for a particular illness. It's up to us to find it.' This principle inspired me, lifted my spirits and gave me the confidence to wage war against autism.

AUTISM ENTAILS FULL-TIME MANAGEMENT FOR THE DOCTOR

A word of advice for any doctor taking on a case like David's: be prepared for micro-management. This isn't the flu or a tummy ache, where there's a once-off consultation and then you don't see your patient until they're sick again – maybe a year later. This is a true partnership between the doctor and the patient's parents.

The same goes for the parent–doctor relationship. If you work against your doctor's advice, you won't achieve the results you're hoping for. It's all about working as a team. The medical professional has to be in partnership with the patient and his or her family.

Defeat Autism Now!

Around this time we stumbled upon the Defeat Autism Now! (DAN!) organisation in the United States.

DAN! was hosting a conference on the treatment of autism in Washington, and we decided that Martin should attend. Excitedly we booked his air ticket and hotel, and made all the necessary arrangements. Martin set off on his journey to the United States hopeful and in anticipation of finding real answers.[2]

The DAN! conference that changed it all

It was at this conference that Martin first met Judy Chinitz, whose son Alex also had autism. Judy took Martin under her wing. Soon he was accepted into Judy's 'Doctor Moms' elite autism treatment unit, earning himself the title of 'Doctor Dad'.

The conference speaker line-up consisted of doctors, nutritionists, neurologists, scientists, biochemists, professors of immunology, gastroenterologists and a host of other medical professionals, all presenting on the treatments of autism. This alone was profound. Coming from South Africa where we had been given no hope, no answers, no treatment plan and nothing much of anything apart from 'goodbye and good luck', things quickly changed. Rising from the depths of gloom and despair, we were suddenly armed with knowledge of autism's underlying causes and treatments – and with hope.

In Washington Martin rubbed shoulders with top scientists and researchers in the field of autism treatment, all of whom presented evidence-based medical solutions to our problem. We had struck gold! No longer were we alone on a dead-end road going nowhere – now we had a plan!

It was also in Washington that Martin first met Dr Jeffrey Bradstreet. After Martin had attended the doctor's presentation, he called me to say: 'I've found our doctor: call his office and book an appointment.'

---

2 DAN!'s work in the United States has now been replaced by the work of the Autism Research Institute.

CHAPTER FIVE

DR JAMES JEFFREY BRADSTREET

Dr Bradstreet (1954–2015) redefined autism. For us he was a beacon of light and the best autism doctor in the world. Years ago, when his son Matthew was diagnosed with autism, Dr Bradstreet began his search for answers. Since then thousands of children worldwide have benefited from his work.

Jeffrey Bradstreet became well known in the autism community as he was able to reverse autism for many children. Admired and respected by his colleagues, he dedicated his life to finding a cure for autism. He was a professor of toxicology, a doctor, a scientist, a researcher and a family friend. Dr Bradstreet was a graduate of the College of Medicine at the University of South Florida and a Fellow of the American Academy of Family Physicians. He published many papers on the treatment of autism and published extensively on the subject of biomedical interventions in autism. Labelled the 'Renaissance man of autism medicine' and an 'avid autism researcher', he'll always be remembered as a hero by the parents of autistic children.

Very few doctors possess the foresight, passion, and determination that Jeff (as we came to call him) displayed. He debunked the archaic approach to autism that looks no further than the initial diagnosis. He looked for the source of symptoms; considered the role of inflammation in the gut and the central nervous system; and studied environmental insults and the role of the immune system. His son Matthew, whom doctors in South Africa would have written off, went on to attend an American college. Jeff proved that autism can be treated.

Dr Bradstreet's magic

Everything Jeff Bradstreet recommended for David worked. He was our go-to person and our lifeline.

One week after Martin returned from Washington, we had our first scheduled Skype consultation with the doctor. Jeff mapped out David's treatment plan and we got busy setting this in motion. We slept easily knowing we were in capable hands. Although distance separated us, he was always available to take our questions and offer advice. His appointment bookings were always back to back, but somehow he managed to find time for us. We consulted him for 11 years. He had his critics and was regarded as controversial by some, but the number of children he saved from autism is testament to his work.

Sadly, Dr Jeff Bradstreet died in 2015. We experienced a profound sense of loss and grief after his passing, as did many other people. Jeff had explored all the options and left no stone unturned to restore health to children suffering from autism and related conditions. He was well aware that he couldn't wait around for the double-blind studies necessary for United States Food and Drug Administration (USFDA) approval; there simply was no time to waste. It can take many years for a drug to get USFDA approval.

As parents drowning in the vast ocean of autism, we couldn't simply tread water waiting for a boat to come around. We had to swim to the shore ourselves. We didn't have the luxury of time. Every second of the day during which our children were sick and wasting away was soul-destroying. I challenge any parent to stand by and accept the cruel and harsh reality of autism that is left untreated.

Many traditional doctors dismissed Jeff's work, lambasting him. Many other scientists were also dismissed when they first released their formulas and discoveries. We need to ask ourselves the question: When does a therapy become science-based? When does it become a cure? Jeff was well aware of his critics. Yet this didn't prevent him from treating children with autism, because his success in treating the disease had far-reaching effects on many lives.

The importance of Dr Jeff Bradstreet's work, as told by Dr Marco Ruggiero

Florence, Italy, 24 June 2013. Dr Jeff Bradstreet, his family and two Italian friends are sitting on the roof of one of the tallest old buildings in the historical birthplace of the Renaissance. It's about 10 pm and the city is celebrating the religious festival of St John, Patron Saint of the city. Palazzo della Signoria, the seat of government of the Medici family whose generosity started the Renaissance, is in the background. One of our Italian friends is a professor of history and human sciences at the University of Florence, and tells us that the Palazzo was accurately built to the millimetre, so its height would be identical to that of the cathedral. This was meant to state, in stone, that the dignity of human reason was not inferior to anything else – the very essence of the spirit of the Renaissance after the dark centuries of the Middle Ages.

At 10 pm the world-famous fireworks start and we're in the privileged position of admiring them with the skyline of the old city as background; it's nothing short of magical. After the fireworks, we imagine how life could have been in the days of the Renaissance when a spirit of freedom was pervading all aspects of life, from art to culture. Our Italian friend however warns us that it wasn't as romantic and idealistic as we now tend to imagine. Centuries after the Renaissance, Galileo, who lived and worked at the observatory of Arcetri that we see in the distance, was condemned to death because of his scientific observations that contradicted the [Church] dogmas. And avoided being burned at the stake only because he chose to renounce his scientific work. Relaxed, we reason that things have changed and that today nobody can be persecuted because of scientific ideas. Our friend, a fine expert in history and the humanities, warns us that history tends to repeat itself ...

Chicago, May 2015. Jeff and I are relaxing after a long day of lectures and scientific meetings. He has learnt of my book, *Your*

Third Brain, the first and only book I have written in my life; and confesses that he has also been asked several times to write a book describing his battles against diseases and prejudices, but has always declined. He asks for my help in writing such a book, sharing our most recent interpretations of the role of the microbiome, this recently discovered mysterious organ. I agree with enthusiasm and begin to record some ideas. A few days later, taking inspiration from some recent observations, I've written a chapter of the book. I reason that the chapter I've written will probably be an appendix of the book. Then, tragedy strikes. Our book will never be written. Only that chapter remains of this project. A chapter that talks about the immortal part of ourselves. A chapter that was later published as an article in a scientific journal: 'The Human Microbiota and the Immune System: Reflections on Immortality'.

MEMORIES

I first met Dr James Jeffrey Bradstreet (Jeff) in Frankfurt, Germany, at the first GcMAF Immunology conference in April 2013. We had exchanged emails in the previous months when Jeff had learnt we were working on the GcMAF molecule (a protein produced by modification of vitamin D-binding protein) *in vitro*. He wished to share with us his experience in treating subjects with autism using the interesting approach that falls under the category of 'immunotherapy'. Since I had acquired my knowledge and training in the scientific-academic medical world of the old continent, with all the formalities that are peculiar of that world, I was struck by his amicability and direct approach. I was impressed that a medical doctor, with his scientific background backed by prestigious peer-reviewed publications, should be so informal and friendly with a colleague he'd never met in person.

I remember one of the first things Jeff told me: 'You've managed to make some enemies in the HIV/AIDS scientific community.' This was in reference to my scientific work with

Prof. Peter Duesberg from Berkeley and our joint publication of a peer-reviewed article challenging the dogmas of the AIDS epidemic. I didn't know at the time that Jeff had also managed to make some powerful enemies in his field of expertise.

A few weeks after our short but intense meeting in Frankfurt, we met Jeff again in Florence, where he'd been invited by an association of parents of autistic children. The organisers had arranged a very intense programme, and I had the honour of helping with the simultaneous translation of his talk from English into Italian. Needless to say the convened parties, who'd come from all over Europe, were astonished to learn about his observations and approach to autism. An approach that had never been heard of before in Italy.

The event went on forever since we couldn't stop the questions. Even though Jeff was clearly exhausted, he continued to answer all the parents' queries until everyone was fully satisfied. Jeff and his wife spent a full week in Florence, and that was when we had the golden opportunity of being invited to watch the fireworks celebrating Florence's Patron Saint, St John, on 24 June from the roof of one of the tallest and oldest buildings of the city with the Palazzo della Signoria as the background. In the course of those few days, Jeff and I spent hours and hours discussing the use of ultrasonography as a harmless and inexpensive tool to study the lesions in the autistic brain and to repair them using the well-documented effects of ultrasound on human neurons and glial cells. It was on that occasion that we decided to modify the programme of our 2013 summer vacations; and to spend a full week with Jeff and his wife in Atlanta, Georgia.

In fact, Jeff decided it was time to put the ultrasonography to the test and invited us to stay with them; the idea was that I would teach Jeff the secrets of the technique I'd just developed to study the evolution of the human brain.

The days following the programme on autism with the parents were among the most intense and amazing of my entire medical-scientific career. I had the opportunity of seeing Jeff visit a number of severely autistic children; and while it's true I taught him some tricks on the use of ultrasonography in detecting the lesions in the brains of autistic children, it's even truer that I was learning a series of lessons on how to deal with the pain and suffering surrounding autism. I learnt more in those few days than in years of medical school, and what I appreciated most was his humanity and sympathy towards that suffering. A humanity and a sympathy that derived from his own experience of being the father of an autistic child.

WORKING TOGETHER TO BREAK THROUGH THE AUTISM BARRIERS

It was then that Jeff and I decided to write a scientific paper describing for the very first time the observation of lesions in the brains of autistic children that might explain the most prominent symptoms of autism. In the following months, Jeff made a series of observations that confirmed our hypothesis and we were eventually able to submit a paper to the prestigious, peer-reviewed journal *Frontiers in Human Neuroscience*. Our article appeared in January 2014.

In October 2013, I had the serendipitous opportunity of meeting Jeff and his wife again, this time in Newport Beach, CA. I'd been invited to Southern California to see a boy with an extreme form of Chronic Fatigue Syndrome; and when I learnt Jeff was attending his clinic in the area, I took the opportunity to see him and his colleagues. From them, I learnt about the preliminary results of an innovative approach termed Transcranial Magnetic Stimulation, a technique aimed at re-establishing brain synchronicity. The results of this work were presented at the AutismOne Conference in Chicago the following year. I remember very well the night we were invited to a barbeque organised by a mutual friend, the founder of a non-profit company with the goal of changing the face of special education and autism. On that occasion Jeff took the opportunity to share with me his worries about the fact that there were many critics of his work, up to the point where someone had felt the need to write a rather derogatory page on him on Wikipedia.

A few weeks later we were together again, this time in Dubai, attending another immunology conference on GcMAF. Regrettably, we couldn't spend much time together. We were so intensely engaged with all those interested in our research that we had little, if any, time left to share our thoughts or enjoy the exotic atmosphere of the Emirates. I remember that Jeff was constantly 'assailed' by parents of autistic children seeking help, and that he never sent them away, every time displaying the sympathy and compassion that all those who knew him experienced.

One night, very late, I came back to the hotel where the conference was hosted after having spoken all day with dignitaries about the possibility of implementing our natural immunotherapy protocol in the Emirates. I was dead tired. I hadn't eaten or drunk all day because of pressing commitments and I was sitting at a table in the hotel restaurant when Jeff came to sympathise with me and share his experiences of dealing with politicians and dignitaries from around the world.

Although we stayed in touch through email and Skype over the following months, it wasn't until May 2014 that we met again, at the AutismOne Conference in Chicago. It was my first time at AutismOne and I had the honour and the privilege of being invited to give the keynote speech together with Jeff. We shared the podium and I presented for the very first time the natural immunotherapy protocol, designated 'the Swiss Protocol'. It was on this occasion that Jeff presented the first results on the therapeutic use of Transcranial Magnetic Stimulation, and the acceptance by the public was simply fantastic. I remember the adrenaline of standing on that podium next to Jeff in front of a competent and attentive audience. Those memories are fixed in my brain and will remain with me as long as I live.

During AutismOne 2014, we found some time to discuss future collaborative projects involving the use of ultrasound in therapy, and the development of an integrated protocol that involved his observation as well as ours. We were also interested in defining the role of the microbiome in the aetiology and pathogenesis of autism and in the interrelationship between the human genes and the genes of the microbiome, and explaining how these relationships could possibly relate to autism. We were still discussing and developing a wealth of projects until the day before his untimely death.

One full year passed before we met again in Chicago at the AutismOne Conference in 2015. In the meantime, I had been planning to move to the United States to start a new enterprise in the field of applied nutrigenomic research, and Jeff had been implementing the use of Transcranial Magnetic Stimulation in his new office. The reunion was joyful and rich with expectations. Jeff lauded my work several times during his talks; and even modified his last talk to accommodate a research project we'd discussed the day before. We were planning to adopt a revolutionary approach and he was so enthusiastic about it that he couldn't refrain from sharing it with the audience at AutismOne. He wanted to merge his protocol with the natural immunotherapy approach and we were thinking of appropriate names for it. We had so many projects and ideas that it would take hundreds of pages to explain them. On the last day of the conference he gave me a big hug, and we promised to meet within the next few weeks.

We actually spoke several times over the phone after the AutismOne Conference: we were working on a collaborative project on ultrasound and human neurons, and thought we were on the brink of some breakthrough observation that might change the whole approach to autism. On the morning of Thursday 18 June 2015, I received a call from him asking me for all the scientific help I could give him. I dropped everything else and immediately sent him all the scientific material I could find capable of supporting his case. I called him back that evening to check that he'd received the material, and he was calm and relaxed. We joked about future developments and he encouraged me to keep on doing the research we'd planned together, since he believed it could change the world of autism. I replied that we were supposed to do it together and that, in my opinion, his actual circumstances were not an obstacle to his work. We left the conversation in a positive mood. The following day, I received the news of his death.

INTERPRETATION OF HOW DR BRADSTREET'S SCIENCE
REDEFINED AUTISM
Dr Bradstreet's science intersected with the science of other researchers/scientific disciplines. [Here I speak] about the ways in which he connected the dots and fitted the pieces together.

Jeff Bradstreet's scientific work was eclectic and multifaceted. His published articles in peer-reviewed journals range from the use of stem cells in treating autism to the role of cannabinoid receptors and the regulation of the epigenome.[3,4]

At the time of his tragic death he had at least two scientific papers submitted for evaluation in major journals and a number of research projects under way. My wife and I are the co-authors with Dr Bradstreet of a paper that was posthumously published in the scientific journal *Frontiers in Neuroscience*, the world's most cited neuroscience journal. This paper sheds light on the role of the immune system inside the brain and opens the way for a radical new approach to autism.

---

3 Siniscalco D, Bradstreet JJ, Cirillo A, Antonucci N. 'The in vitro GcMAF effects on endocannabinoid system transcriptionomics, receptor formation, and cell activity of autism-derived macrophages.' *J Neuroinflammation.* 2014 Apr 17;11:78. doi: 10.1186/1742-2094-11-78. PMID: 24739187. Available at https://www.ncbi.nlm.nih.gov/pubmed/24739187, accessed 15 April 2019

4 National Human Genome Research Institute, University of California, Los Angeles: 'UCLA-led team uncovers critical new clues about what goes awry in brains of people with autism'. Available at https://www.genome.gov/27532724/epigenomics-fact-sheet/, accessed 11 April 2019

Although each one of the papers published by Jeff is worth a commentary, describing its importance in the field of autism diagnosis and treatment, here I briefly outline something that has not been published yet. In fact, in the days preceding his death, we were working on a hypothesis that could have dramatically changed the very conception of autism and of several other neurological and psychiatric disorders.

This hypothesis of ours starts with some rather provocative statements: that we have three brains – the brain inside our head, a second brain consisting of the neurons in the wall of the gastrointestinal tract, and a non-human third brain made up of billions of microbes constituting the newly discovered organ termed the 'microbiome'; that the brain inside our head (the 'first brain') is under the control of the third brain; that autism results from the malfunctioning of the microbiome; and that we will be able to restore the working of the first brain by correcting this malfunction.

As a matter of fact, there are hundreds of scientific articles describing how the composition of the microbial environment in our bodies, and principally in the gut, is responsible for our mood, behaviour and capacity to cope with stress. Some articles explicitly state that the microbes manipulate us to increase their own fitness, whereas other articles propose the use of psychobiotics to treat mental illnesses such as depression. In sum, there is solid scientific evidence demonstrating that our supposed free will is not free at all, but is controlled by the microbes inside us.

The relationship between autism and the microbiome is not a new concept. The University of Utah, in a tutorial describing the role of the microbiome in a variety of diseases, clearly states:

> The search for the cause of autism has turned up several weak genetic links and many suspected environmental triggers. Now researchers have learnt that microbes may also be involved. A few small studies have shown that children with autism have different microbes living

in their intestines than children without the disorder. This difference could be explained by the often picky eating habits of autistic children. Or the difference could be a side effect of an underlying genetic or environmental trigger – autistic children commonly have gastro-intestinal problems. Still, the connection is intriguing. The causes of autism are varied and complex and the same measures may prevent the disease in some – but not in others. By learning about the connection between autism and microbes, we have the potential to find more ways to fight the disorder.

We can further elaborate that the so-called 'picky eating habits of autistic children' could be the result of the manipulation of these eating habits by the microbes themselves.[5]

Moreover, quite recently on Yahoo, a revealing article supporting these notions was published describing 'The link between gut bacteria and your kid's behaviour' (see References list below).

All in all, it seems there is general consensus that autism and altered composition and functioning of the microbiome are strictly interrelated. However, a comprehensive hypothesis and an integrated approach have not yet been proposed, and Jeff and I were working on exactly these issues in the days preceding his death. We had come to believe autism was the consequence of alterations of the third brain. As such, it could be treated by targeting this organ rather than treating the symptoms. In fact, it's very well known that autism involves alterations in the digestive and immune systems; but what had not been envisaged was the notion that the digestive and immune systems, as well as human brains, are all under the control of the non-human third brain constituted by the microbiome.

We were on the brink of a revolutionary approach that, by

---

5 Alcock J, Maley CC, Aktipis CA. 'Is eating behavior manipulated by the gastrointestinal microbiota? Evolutionary pressures and potential mechanisms.' *Bioessays*. 2014 Oct;36(10):940-9. doi: 10.1002/bies.201400071. Epub 2014 Aug 8. PMID: 25103109. PMCID: PMC4270213. Available at https://www.ncbi.nlm.nih.gov/pubmed/25103109, accessed 15 April 2019

targeting the microbiome itself, could have solved all the issues associated with autism at once. If we were able to demonstrate our hypothesis, the definition of autism itself would have changed. In fact, instead of talking of a neurodevelopmental, or behavioural, or neuropsychiatric, or immunological disorder, we could have defined autism as a disease of the microbiome – a disease of a non-human organ that had gone undetected until recently. And, most importantly, of an organ we now know how to repair, meaning a disease that could be cured once and for all. It was no coincidence that the last talk by Jeff at AutismOne was titled: 'How close are we to an autism cure?'

THE SCIENCE EXPLAINED

Recent science is shining light on the real physiological factors underlying the diagnostic label 'autism'.

On the very last day of the AutismOne Conference in 2015, Jeff told me about a scientific collaborative project that he cherished and wished to realise in the shortest possible time, in order to develop a joint protocol for the treatment of autism and complex disorders. As a matter of fact, even though Jeff's fame is inextricably linked to his innovative approach to autism spectrum disorders, he was a talented medical doctor who treated a number of pathologies – ranging from cancer through HIV infection and Chronic Fatigue Syndrome. Consistent with this approach, his blog, which was both scientifically sound and constantly updated, read: 'Hope for complex health issues'. Therefore, it was in his interest to merge the protocol that I had developed with his own approach. The idea was to develop a protocol that could target the common cellular and molecular mechanisms that are at the basis of a variety of diseases.

Jeff's tragic death prevented the development of such a collaborative protocol. Nevertheless, we had time to share some ideas, which I wish to impart in the following pages.

The Protocol was to be developed on the basis of more than 30 years' scientific research in the fields of molecular biology, neuroscience and oncology. Its intent was to provide the immune system with strong support; and to counteract some of the effects of chronic conditions and ageing by reconstituting an organ, the microbiome, that had eluded the attention of the medical/scientific community for millennia.

We decided to develop the Protocol on the basis of the new discoveries concerning the microbiome, and also on the principles of the *Allgemeine Pathologie* (German for 'General Pathology'). This European medical discipline, which I brought to Jeff's attention, focuses on the common characteristics shared by different diseases. In fact, although diseases have different causes (aetiology) and different ways of progressing (their 'pathogenesis'), they share core common features at the cellular and molecular levels. The Protocol that Jeff and I were discussing was to be developed to target those common features, so it could be applied to the maintenance of good health as well as the treatment of a variety of diseases including autism and cancer.

In many instances, the Protocol could not have been considered an alternative to conventional methods of addressing diseases. Rather, it represented a complementary approach that aimed to maximise the therapeutic effects of conventional approaches while at the same time reducing the side effects of those approaches. This would be done by reconstituting the microbiome – an organ that participates in the development and functions of all other organs and systems of the human body. Therefore, we believed that the Protocol could be implemented in conjunction with any other type of therapeutic approach, whether conventional or complementary.

Our idea of the Protocol was based on three tenets: establishing a diet that helped the microbiome; reconstituting the immune system; and reconstituting the human healthy core microbiome.

An organ that has been ignored for millennia

According to the National Institutes of Health (NIH) that is running the Human Microbiome Project (HMP) in the United States, the typical healthy person is inhabited by billions of microbes and each person's microbiome is unique. That is, two people may have very different microbial communities but still both be healthy. However, the researchers found that despite this uniqueness, the presence of certain communities of microbes could be used to predict certain individual characteristics. For example, whether you were breastfed as an infant and even your level of education could be predicted based on microbial communities across varying body sites. The analysis also showed that microbial communities from varying body sites on the same individual were predictive for other microbial communities. For example, gut communities could be predicted by examining the oral community, even though these communities are vastly different from each other. According to the NIH, this microbiome-based approach will help pave the way for future studies that will be able to use microbial communities as a basis for the personalising of therapies and possibly to assess an individual's risk for certain diseases.

The concept of the microbiome emerged shortly after the characterisation of the human genome. In fact, the suffix 'ome' was derived from the information that was gathered from studying the human genome.

The studies on the human genome demonstrated that the genetic information for humans is encoded in about 20 000 genes. These are responsible for the synthesis and functions of all our proteins; and hence of our cells and, ultimately, our organs. However, the HMP also demonstrated that total microbial cells found in association with humans may exceed the total number of cells making up the human body by a factor of ten to one and, perhaps more strikingly, that the total number of genes associated with the human microbiome may exceed the total number of human genes by a factor of a hundred to one. The organisms thought to be found in the human microbiome are generally categorised as bacteria (the majority), members of domain Archaea, yeasts, and single-celled eukaryotes. Other organisms encountered there are various helminths, parasites and viruses, the latter including viruses that infect cellular microbiome organisms.

Weighing about 2 kg, the microbiome plays a fundamental role in the development of all other organs, as well as in their function throughout the phases of human life, from birth to old age.

According to the University of Utah:

> As researchers learn more about the microbes that keep us healthy, we are coming to understand how subtle imbalances in our microbial populations can also cause disease—and how restoring the balance may lead to cures. Our new understanding may lead to more focused and effective treatments. Unlike modern antibiotics, which kill good microbes along with the bad, new drugs may kill only harmful bacteria while leaving the friendly ones alone. Others may nurture friendly bacteria, helping them out-compete the harmful ones.

Therefore, the goal of the Protocol that Jeff and I were developing was fully consistent with the above statements as it was precisely intended to restore the balance of the microbiome and to nurture friendly bacteria, helping them to out-compete the harmful ones.

THE NEED FOR THE RIGHT NUTRITION

The human microbiome needs appropriate nutrition in order to maintain its properties and a healthy microbiome is essential for proper nutrition. It's even more important than food itself in maintaining a good state of nutrition. In fact, a study examining identical twins, one twin undernourished and the other not, revealed that although the twins had the same genes and ate the same food, they had different gut microbiota.

Jeff and I knew very well that most autistic subjects are somehow malnourished and we found that the best type of nutrition to maintain a healthy microbiome is rich in proteins and poor in carbohydrates. It's well known that a high-protein/low-carbohydrate diet is useful in almost all chronic conditions.

Consistent with this approach, and before I met Jeff, my research group had been working for about 30 years on the role of glycolysis in carcinogenesis and other human diseases. We published 13 papers on the role of the by-products of glycolysis (diacylglycerol) in cancer; and also in neurodegenerative diseases, chronic kidney disease and cardiovascular disease.

We believed that subjects should be on a high-protein, high-fat and anti-inflammatory diet, with a significant reduction in the consumption of carbohydrates. It was important for such a status to be achieved in a progressive way, without withdrawing carbohydrates too abruptly and incurring weight loss and, in particular, the loss of (lean) muscle mass. Our nutritional plan was based on an increasing number of data demonstrating the usefulness of these diets in a variety of metabolic diseases such as obesity, metabolic syndrome, diabetes, cancer and autism. Jeff and I were convinced that low-carb/high-protein nutrition was important in achieving the best responses from the neuro-protective/immunotherapeutic approach described below.

When the tragedy struck, we were on the verge of implementing an integrative Protocol that, in our opinion, had the potential to be useful in a variety of conditions ranging from autism to cancer.

THE IMMUNE SYSTEM AND RECONSTITUTION OF THE
(HUMAN) HEALTHY CORE MICROBIOME
According to the University of Utah, autism, cancer, depression,

diabetes, malnutrition and autoimmune diseases are just some of the health conditions that involve our microbes; and for which our Protocol, encompassing the use of live probiotics, could have proven useful. In addition to reconstituting the human microbiome, most of the microbial strains contained in our approach show, in and of themselves, beneficial effects in a variety of conditions. Their mechanisms of action at the molecular level converge in stimulating and rebalancing the immune system and in promoting other health effects. For example, we and others demonstrated the role of macrophage activation in the treatment of a number of conditions. Interestingly, one of the strains we used, *Lactobacillus Rhamnosus*, also activates macrophages, thus converging on the same immune-stimulatory pathway with a synergistic effect.

In addition, some of the probiotic microbial strains that we envisaged are associated with the endogenous production of neurotransmitters and second messengers that are known to rebalance and improve neurological functions and neuronal connectivity. In fact, there is increasing evidence suggesting an interaction between the intestinal microbiota, the gut, and the central nervous system – in what is recognised as the microbiome–gut–brain axis or 'the third brain'. For example, recent data on *Lactobacillus Rhamnosus* suggest that these microbes can modulate the GABAergic system; and may therefore have beneficial effects in the treatment of depression and anxiety.

To sum up, therefore, we intended to design a natural, nutrition-based immunotherapeutic approach with the objective of exploiting the intriguing opportunity of developing unique microbial-based strategies for the adjunctive treatment of stress-related psychiatric and neurodegenerative disorders as well as autism spectrum disorders.

In addition, given the interest Jeff had in the therapeutic use of ultrasound and on the basis of our paper published in *Frontiers in Human Neuroscience*, we'd decided to explore the therapeutic potential of such a technique. In fact, based on some clinical observations, we postulated a synergy between transcranial ultrasonography (TUS) and the Protocol, with the ultimate goal of maximising its neuro-protective, immunotherapeutic effects.

Moreover, the development of a non-invasive, anatomically targeted method for the controlled modulation of regional brain activity offered a new opportunity in creating a wide range of applications for the treatment of neurologic and neuropsychiatric disorders. TUS-mediated modulation of neuronal activity opens new avenues of clinical applications for the treatment of various neurological and psychiatric illnesses.

According to Prof. Stuart Hameroff at the University of Arizona, TUS acts via intra-neuronal microtubules, which apparently resonate in TUS megahertz range, and Jeff and I hypothesised that TUS might help us nanosize bioactive molecules inside the affected areas of the brain toward which the TUS were directed. Based on our experience, we thought that TUS might be applied through the temporal acoustic window on the same side of the head as a unilateral neurological lesion; or through both acoustic windows if the lesions were bilateral. By using accurate settings we might visualise the cerebral cortex, thus indicating that the ultrasound waves were reaching the grey matter. We found that most regions of the brain could be accessed through the temporal acoustic window. In addition, and maybe more importantly, we hypothesised that the effects of the molecules administered as part of the Protocol would be significantly amplified by nanosizing these molecules in proximity of the lesions that we had described in our seminal paper in *Frontiers in Human Neuroscience*.

REFERENCES

Bioessays. 2014 Oct;36(10):940-9. Is eating behavior manipulated by the gastrointestinal microbiota? Evolutionary pressures and potential mechanisms. Alcock J, Maley CC, Aktipis CA

Brain Stimul. 2013 May;6(3):409-15. Transcranial ultrasound (TUS) effects on mental states: a pilot study. Hameroff S, Trakas M, Duffield C, Annabi E, Gerace MB, Boyle P, Lucas A, Amos Q, Buadu A, Badal JJ

Front Hum Neurosci. 2014 Jan 15;7:934. doi: 10.3389/fnhum.2013.00934. eCollection 2014. A new methodology of viewing extra-axial fluid and cortical abnormalities in children with autism via transcranial ultrasonography. Bradstreet JJ, Pacini S, Ruggiero M

Front Neurosci. 2015 Dec 22;9:485. doi: 10.3389/fnins.2015.00485. eCollection 2015.

Commentary: Structural and functional features of central nervous system lymphatic vessels. Bradstreet JJ, Ruggiero M, Pacini S

Front Pediatr. 2014 Jun 30;2:69. doi: 10.3389/fped.2014.00069. eCollection 2014. Potential therapeutic use of the ketogenic diet in autism spectrum disorders. Napoli E, Dueñas N, Giulivi C

http://commonfund.nih.gov/hmp/programhighlights#biome

https://www.yahoo.com/news/the-link-between-gut-bacteria-and-your-kids-122912819857.html

Ital J Anat Embryol. 2011;116(2):73-92. AIDS since 1984: no evidence for a new, viral epidemic – not even in Africa. Duesberg PH, Mandrioli D, McCormack A, Nicholson JM, Rasnick D, Fiala C, Koehnlein C, Bauer HH, Ruggiero M

Ital J Anat Embryol. 2013;118(3):241-55.Transcranial sonography: a technique for the study of the temporal lobes of the human and non-human primate brain. Ruggiero M, Magherini S, Fiore MG, Chiarelli B, Morucci G, Branca JJ, Gulisano M, Pacini S

Neurogastroenterol Motil. 2013 Sep;25(9):713-19. doi: 10.1111/nmo.12198. Melancholic microbes: a link between gut microbiota and depression? Dinan TG, Cryan JF

Proc. Natl. Acad. Sci. U. S. A. 2011 Sep;108(38):16050-16055. doi: 10.1073/pnas.1102999108. Ingestion of *Lactobacillus* strain regulates emotional behavior and central GABA receptor expression in a mouse via the vagus nerve. Bravo JA, Forsythe P, Chew MV, Escaravage E, Savignac HM, Dinan TG, Bienenstock J, Cryan JF

CHAPTER SIX

AUTISM TREATMENT 101

The gut–brain connection in autism

One of the causes of David's crying, developmental delay, discomfort and pain was his gut. He couldn't tell us what the problem was – all he had was his crying. We'd often find him hanging upside down over a chair, trying to put pressure on his aching tummy to relieve the sharp piercing pains penetrating his body. Contrary to the common assumption that he required deep pressure, brushing, and vestibular and proprioceptive input, he actually desperately needed expert medical attention to treat his gut.

His loose bowel movements continued, varying from four to ten foul-smelling stools a day. We now know that this is a common condition in children with autism; that David's cries were undoubtedly coming from the discomfort and pain in his tummy; and that his pale skin and the dark rings around his eyes were all indicators of a deeper, underlying gut problem. Looking back now, I'm horrified by the fact that the neurologist I consulted in those early days prescribed Risperdal. I was given psychiatric medication to treat a child suffering from a bowel disorder! The test results available ought also to have made it clear to this specialist that the problem was much more severe than mere toddler's diarrhoea as diagnosed by our local paediatrician, who, at the time, didn't link David's developmental delays to autism or make any gut–brain connection.

David undergoes a colonoscopy

We consulted with Dr Arthur Krigsman, a reputable New York-based paediatric gastroenterologist specialising in autism. He recommended that we make arrangements for David to have a colonoscopy and a scan via ingested capsule camera. These interventions would hopefully give us the important information we needed to ascertain what was causing David's distended belly and irritable bowel. We'd always felt that David would start to develop if only we could get his gut under control: no child in constant pain can learn properly.

Dr Krigsman urged us either to fly to New York with David so he could conduct a colonoscopy or to set up a colonoscopy in South Africa. There are very few paediatric gastroenterologists in South Africa. After we had consulted a local paediatric gastroenterologist who casually dismissed us, confident in her view that there was no link between autism and gut health, we decided to consult a gastroenterologist specialising in adults.

Martin met with the doctor to explain our son's case and to ask him whether he would be prepared to scope David. He agreed, and proceeded to order special paediatric equipment from a country overseas. The day before the colonoscopy, David had to drink the usual preparation everyone takes prior to the procedure. It was difficult to get him to drink the unpleasant-smelling, bitter yellow liquid that would cause his bowel to empty in preparation for the next day.

We arrived at the hospital at 6 am, ready for the procedure. Martin and I felt great trepidation and were aware of the hollow in the pit of our stomachs. After a nervous conversation with the anaesthetist, who assured us that David would cope well with being put to sleep, we watched our son being wheeled into theatre. Martin and I stood outside the door. I could hear the heart monitor from where we were standing; and I remember that its beeping stopped for a few seconds. Anxiously, I called a nurse over to ask her why it had gone quiet, but she promised us all was well. Eventually, the gastroenterologist appeared from behind the closed door and told us he'd managed to secure biopsies from all the areas of David's gut, including the ileum and the colon. He had not seen any signs of inflammation, he added. I was quite disappointed he hadn't found anything wrong, as I'd hoped the procedure would lead us to the discovery of a cause for David's symptoms – and to possible treatment. However, we knew that the biopsies might provide more information.

Waiting for the results from the biopsies

We sent the samples both to our local South African laboratory and to Dr Krigsman's laboratory in the United States. We'd pre-arranged for the biopsies to be preserved in wax blocks so they could be shipped overseas for testing. Once again, Martin took on the task of driving our precious cargo to the FedEx head office close to the airport.

I called Judy Chinitz and was relieved to hear that the inflammation so often found in children with autism can be microscopic, which might explain why the gastroenterologist, who was used to treating adults, had not found any signs of it while performing the colonoscopy. We eagerly awaited the test results.

Two weeks later, our local laboratory's results revealed 'irregular molecular structure' in the biopsies of the ileum and the colon. The report stated that the laboratory had never before seen this in a child of David's age, and didn't know what to call it. It suggested we wait to hear what the laboratory in the United States had to say.

That laboratory did have something more to say, and it was crucial. In a telephonic appointment, Dr Krigsman revealed that its tests had uncovered the presence of Nodular Lymphoid Hyperplasia (NLH) in David's samples. NLH refers to chronic inflammation of the colorectum, small bowel and stomach; and is a condition frequently reported in children with ASD. It is treated with Colazal (balsalazide disodium) capsules and sometimes with Prednisone.

The microscopic inflammation had been confirmed. The source of David's ill health had been exposed, and we were finally beginning to discern the true nature of autism.

I decide to increase the dose

Working in consultation with Dr Bradstreet, Dr Krigsman prescribed cortisone in the form of Prednisone. We began introducing the drug but saw no change after the first few days. We were on a continuous roller coaster. Only when we doubled the dose did David's gut start to heal. It took courage to administer such a high dose of the drug. As I reluctantly measured out the new dose, I was petrified of what this could do to my precious baby, who was already fighting so hard to exist. But we had no choice: we doubled the dose. Then, for the first time in over four years, David started to have a single, properly formed, bowel movement a day.

This was definitely a major breakthrough that brought us some relief. However, like any other medical intervention, Prednisone has side effects: David was irritable and couldn't sleep, and the medicine caused his yeast issue to flare up. We gave him anti-fungal medication and this calmed the side effects. Over time his gut health improved and we saw positive changes that affected his development favourably. For a while I could breathe again, felt a little like eating and slept through the night. I felt a flicker of hope that we'd be able to pull David from the mire of autism that had stolen him from us.

A brand-new diet

We stopped giving David a bottle and put him on a gluten-free, casein-free (GF/CF), soya-free and sugar-free diet when he was 22 months old. David had drawn comfort from his bottle, and it wasn't easy to take away from him the one thing he had relied on to soothe himself. It was a very sudden change for him and a trying time for us. Following the GF/CF diet required enormous commitment and endurance, especially in South Africa where it isn't easy to find satisfactory food alternatives. Gluten-free means no grains at all, including no spelt.

Casein-free means no dairy, and also no products containing casein. Years later, when I visited Austin, Texas, and had a life-changing experience at a 'wholefoods store' there, I realised why Judy Chinitz could never understand our complaints about the horrid diet we bravely tried to follow.

The American wholefoods store looked like a massive warehouse laden with rows and rows and rows of organic, sugar-free, soya-free, gluten-free, casein-free and other products that not only looked fantastic but also tasted delicious. I was like a child visiting Disneyland for the first time.

I can describe the early years of this diet in only one way – gruelling and depressing. Previously, David had enjoyed shopping with me at a specific supermarket, and had always looked forward to a red sugar lollipop that was soothing for him. Once we started the diet, it meant no more lollipops and no birthday parties. To this day, I'm not fond of kids' birthday parties. I decided that if David couldn't have a lollipop, I wouldn't put him or me in a position in which I had to deny him what he so dearly loved as a treat. I didn't shop at that supermarket for a year; and can confidently report that David didn't have a single grain of sugar during that time. I lost a huge amount of weight when David was on this diet. His meal options were limited, and I couldn't enjoy food while he was deprived of all the things I perceived to be delicious and good to eat.

When we started the diet, I woke up on the first morning in a panic and shook Martin's shoulder to wake him. Tearfully, I shared my concerns about what I was going to feed David when he woke at 6 am. There was no formula bottle to quell his hunger pangs, and breakfast was no longer a simple task of putting a slice of bread in the toaster or giving him a bowl of cereal.

It wasn't easy to wrap my head around the idea that cereal or toast would no longer be an option for breakfast. Instead, David had to get used to avocado, gluten-free pancakes, and mince and rice for breakfast. There were no exciting snacks and no treats. I made thick chicken soup and beef soup, and froze them in special glass containers. I'd been a vegetarian for years and initially it wasn't easy to make chicken soup. I learnt to use my sense of smell to tell me whether I'd been successful in bringing together the hand-selected items I combined for his soup.

We desperately wanted David to get better and develop, and knew we had no choice but to stick regimentally to this diet. Because his gut flora had been destroyed from the early use of antibiotics, he was struggling to break down his food and derive nutrients from it. Soup is nutritious and wholesome, and luckily remained a very popular item on David's food menu for years. After all this practice, I have to say, my chicken soup today is exceptional!

It's important to remember that every child with autism is different; and that tweaking the diet to suit and benefit your child takes much trial and error. However, many parents have reported great benefits to their children from sticking to the GF/CF diet.

Although the diet helped a great deal, David's test results continued to show yeast and bacterial overgrowth for a very long time. It took years of anti-fungal treatment and treatment for bacteria (clostridia) to address the bad bugs in his intestinal tract.

Other ways of tackling autism as a medical illness

As we grew in the belief that autism was a medical illness, we looked for other things to do to help our son. David had been labelled as autistic, but the professionals we had consulted in the early years had not thought of looking at the underlying causes of his condition. In general, by not describing autism as a serious but treatable medical illness, the medical profession has failed the parents of autistic children. There's no reason simply to accept a diagnosis of autism as cast in stone. Or for medical professionals to view autism as just a case of 'neurodiversity'.

AUTISM'S TYPICALLY IMPAIRED IMMUNE SYSTEM

We decided that, in conjunction with settling David's gut, we would tackle his malfunctioning immune system. Research has shown that children with autism have serious abnormalities in the functioning of their immune system; and that if you want to bring your child back from autism, you have to repair and maintain that system. Numerous published studies and papers by highly respected medical professionals worldwide are available on this topic, reinforcing the empirical evidence.

Neuroinflammation and encephalitis (inflammation of the brain) are common in children with autism. Treating the dysregulated immune system is essential to restoring brain function and health. Autism is in fact an 'auto-immune encephalitis' in which the dysfunctional immune system causes brain inflammation. Therefore, treating David's immune system might lead to the reversal of his autism symptoms. On this topic also, there are published papers backing the evidence.

IMPAIRED DETOXIFICATION AND GLUTATHIONE:
GETTING RID OF TOXINS

Our bodies are designed to remove the toxins we're exposed to every day. Children with autism may have an impaired detoxification system, which means that their bodies may not be able to remove toxins adequately. There are many studies showing the potential role of toxic metals in autism.

David's lab reports showed high levels of toxicity and low levels of glutathione (GSH), a common finding in autism. GSH is the garbage truck of the brain, picking up all the toxins. Children with autism are genetically low in GSH.

Both Dr McCandless and Dr Bradstreet encouraged us to administer intravenous GSH to David. Chelation was also recommended, to remove the toxins identified in the samples we sent to the US labs for analysis. These results revealed high levels of mercury, lead, aluminium and arsenic. Sources of mercury include dental fillings, fish such as tuna, and vaccines containing the preservative thimerosal. The symptoms of mercury poisoning are similar to those of autism and include:

❏ gastrointestinal abnormalities
❏ cognitive impairment
❏ delayed speech
❏ issues in sensory processing
❏ toe-walking
❏ self-injurious behaviours
❏ stereotypical behaviours.[6]

6 Shaw, William. 2008, third edition. *Biological Treatments for Autism and PDD.* USA: Sunflower Press

The subdued agony of the drip

David was three years old when we started the search for a doctor to help us administer infusions. We had a few agonising failed attempts by doctors and nurses who couldn't find a vein. I stood by David's side watching as the needle penetrated his soft baby skin. I witnessed the tears roll down his cheeks and heard his frantic screams of pain and panic. I felt helpless, afraid and traumatised. Every time the needle pierced his skin, his vein would jump or the blood wouldn't tap to allow the doctor to insert the IV. I held my breath in anticipation of the next needle. David kicked and screamed as we held him down on the bed. His big eyes fixed on my gaze, pleading with me to make them stop. After numerous attempts we left the doctor's room in a dreadful state, not having managed to administer the IV treatment. Anger, sadness and despair set in. All we had to show for our efforts the next day was blue marks all over his arms that reminded us of the day before. We'd failed and hit rock bottom.

That evening, though, there was an unexpected knock at the door. Martin's business partner and dear friend Bernie Sher had heard about our ordeal and come over to offer support. He sat down with us at the dining room table and listened to us as we recounted the horrific events of the day before. Martin was adamant we'd never attempt IV treatment again, as he couldn't bear to put his baby through such trauma. Bernie encouraged us not to give up and to find a way. He dried our tears and lifted our spirits. He offered us a shoulder to cry on when we needed it most and gave us confidence that everything would work out.

When Bernie left, we started to brainstorm. Martin came up with the idea of going to CHOC, the foundation that treats children with cancer. Surely they had trained nurses who could find veins in young children easily?

A WELCOME ANSWER

We were referred to the Paediatric Oncology Department at the Charlotte Maxeke Hospital, and scheduled an appointment with the departmental head. The day before our appointment, Martin and I prepared the documents and paperwork in support of our request. It's never easy to ask for a favour, and there was so much at stake ...

Armed with books and files, Martin met with them to explain David's case history and why we needed their help. It took strength of character and a vast amount of determination to secure the treatments we needed. I hovered anxiously near the phone, waiting for Martin's call to let me know what their decision was. After listening to our case history and supporting argument for infusions, they agreed to the treatments. Their doctors are accomplished oncologists, and for five years they helped us by inserting David's infusions, including GSH and IVIG (intravenous immunoglobulin).

The nurses and doctors at the paediatric oncology ward showed us remarkable care, empathy and compassion. On the first day, we were shown around the ward and David was allocated a bed. We'd wake early at home in order to arrive in time for the doctors to insert the infusions before they did ward rounds. I'd sleep uneasily the night before in anticipation of the next day. I'd pack a bag with toys and food and anything else I could think of that would keep David occupied and distracted. I'd wake him, dress him and bundle him into the car. Once we'd parked our car in the parking lot we had to walk some way to the lift that took us up to the seventh-floor paediatric ward. It was old and shaky, and I was always concerned about getting stuck.

THE INFUSIONS ARE SUCCESSFULLY ADMINISTERED
The oncologists were highly skilled in finding a vein. Initially, we wrapped David firmly in a blanket with only one arm free, but he sensed that he could trust the oncologist and very early on it was no longer necessary to wrap him. David soon crawled into their hearts. They hardly ever pricked him more than once, and we became confident about their ability to insert the infusion so quickly that David felt minimal pain or distress. We'd found a way and felt pleased we were at last able to administer the treatments.

For the first year we went for the infusions once a week and then stretched the treatment to two weeks apart. GSH accelerated David's healing and we experienced moments of hope as a result of improved eye contact, receptive language and a boy who was more connected and no longer vacant in the

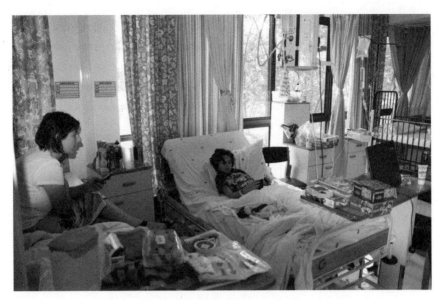

David in the cancer ward

physical body that imprisoned his soul. I'd hold David's hand tightly on the way down and we'd run back to the car to escape the hospital. The image of the liquid in the IV bag slowly dripping into his veins is still etched in my memory. Every infusion was an accomplishment.

Mixed emotions on the cancer ward

Experiencing the paediatric oncology ward evoked mixed emotions in me. I watched the young children with cancer receive their treatments. I remember fixing my gaze on an exchange between one of the moms and her three-year-old daughter who was receiving treatment. While her mother lovingly propped up the cushion behind her back and sat her up for a few sips of apple juice, adjusting the beanie on her bald head, the little girl spoke to her. I eavesdropped on their conversation for some time. She could tell her mom how she felt; that she was thirsty and needed another pillow; and that she wanted her mom to read her a story. I was overcome with a deep sense of sadness and anger. I also adjusted the cushion behind David to make him comfortable during the infusion and caringly gave him

71

sips of water to quench his thirst – but the difference was that he couldn't ask for these things. He couldn't tell me about his pain or how he was feeling or what he wanted. He didn't ask me to read him a story and I walked around the ward in the deepest grief imaginable. I no longer thought cancer was the worst-case scenario. At least the mom who was fighting cancer had the luxury of engaging with her child.

Over the months I became immune to the fact that we were visiting the paediatric oncology ward. I had thought about it deeply and envied the parents of the cancer patients. Even though their children faced a life-threatening illness, they were sharing experiences with their children and making memories to treasure. We had no special bag of memories; and very little to show apart from special diets, medical treatments and memories of David's cries and screams. I could only look at David and try to imagine why he was smiling or why he was wearing a particular facial expression. How could I explain why I grieved for a child I hadn't lost?

My reaction may seem harsh, but these emotions are by no means rare among the parents of autistic children who are unable to acquire language. I will let another mother, who took to expressing her feelings through a blog, tell it like it is for so many parents of children who cannot speak:

As I sat on the bench in a public park, the tears came easily. Watching little toddlers peddling trikes and mothers chatting to babies. Seeing pre-school children laughing and chatting as they wheeled around the water on their brightly coloured scooters.

It has been building for a while.

The night before last it was anger and hurt as a friend shared how her 14 month old was defiantly talking back when they were trying to get her to bed. I wanted to scream and say 'but she understands! But she talks!' Instead I mourned silently.

The world goes on while I grieve for a child I haven't lost.

It's a pain that is very different from other pains. I know the pain of not having children. I know the pain of losing a yet-to-be-born baby. I know the pain of losing someone very close. I know that feeling of despair and anger and hopelessness.

People understand when they know you have loved and lost. But how do you explain that you are grieving a child you haven't lost?

I get to read to my son. I get to bathe him and dress him and kiss him. I hear him laugh when I tickle him and get to push him on the swings at the park. He goes to school. He'll watch a video sometimes. And yet he is lost.

I have yet to hear his voice. I grieve for the conversations we will never have. I grieve the fact I will never hear him sing or shout or chat with friends like those little ones in the park. I grieve for the fact I will never hear him tell me a joke or talk to me about his day at school. I grieve for the loss of never hearing him whisper 'I love you'. I can only dream about what his little voice may sound like, how it may have grown in depth and tone as he aged, what sort of accent he may have had or how he may have pronounced the names of people he knew. A part of him will never be. And I feel the loss and pain of that.

I grieve for all the milestones I've missed and may never have with him. As I watched a mum bend down to hold her son's hand today to help him walk, I thought about how much she takes for granted. Her little one was not much over a year old and yet he confidently held her hand to take some steps. By the time my child did anything like this he was tall enough that I had no need to bend; and his hands were nothing like as tiny as her son's. I have skipped the toilet training, the bike riding, the learning to read and write, the school plays, the attending clubs and the having friends. I have been robbed of things others take for granted and that should be part of normal childhood. There is a loss and a sadness for times that might have been but will never be.

There is sadness that I cannot walk him to school or that he cannot go to school with his twin sister. There is pain relying on others to tell me about his day when I should hear it from him. There is heartbreak watching the neighbour's child of the same age jump on a trampoline [while] my son cannot balance on one leg let alone jump. There's a lump in my throat when people ask what my child wants for Christmas and he still plays with baby toys at [the age of] almost seven. We have never experienced the Tooth Fairy with him, and he has no concept of Santa Claus. [Neither does he] choose his own clothes [or have] the ability to dress himself. He has never said 'Mummy can I have' or gone in a strop because he cannot go out to play. He has no friends his own age and doesn't get invited to parties.

He is here, but to many he isn't.

I have a son. He is my pride and joy. I am so proud of everything he does. But I still grieve for him, for the things he will never achieve and the experiences he will never have. And I grieve for myself as a parent when I see a world of parenting I can only ever dream about.

As I sat on the bench in a public park the tears came easily; tears of heartache and anger, tears of frustration and pain.

It's all part of the journey. Before I can move on, I need to grieve for the loss. And grieving takes time. So please forgive me and support me. Life goes on and I understand that. I have no bitterness at that. But sometimes those tears are needed. Bear with me as I grieve for a child I haven't lost.

Miriam Gwynne – Special needs blogger – www.faithmummy.wordpress.com

Some heavy sacrifices, Barney the purple dinosaur and glimpses of hope

Martin had to work and often travelled overseas. It was very painful to leave Eli at home for hours at a time while I was at the hospital with David. I was unsettled all the time, knowing I wasn't there for Eli at this very important time of life, when a baby needs his mother.

Ultimately, it became my responsibility to take David for the infusions. Just like David, I was alive but not really there. The infusions took hours. Keeping David occupied for long periods of time proved challenging. I used to walk him around the ward and up and down the corridors, carefully wheeling the IV bag he was hooked up to behind us. It reminded me of the shackled prisoners receiving medical treatment whom I'd seen earlier on my way up to the ward. There was no escape.

There was one saving grace. As he had when he was younger, David enjoyed watching movies about Barney the purple dinosaur, and we'd play these movies over and over and over. Without Barney, I doubt we'd have survived the infusions and the agonisingly long hours we spent at the hospital. David was glued to Barney and Barney soaked up the six hours it took to infuse the IVIG.

We had hoped IVIG would make it easier for David to produce vocal language. After nine months of infusions, David made noticeable improvements in his overall health. He became more alert, his understanding improved and he became able to discriminate between objects, learning different object labels. This was a breakthrough.

Chelation

In order to remove the heavy metals identified in the samples sent to the US laboratories, we started chelation. This is the method used to remove mercury and other heavy metals and toxins, including lead, arsenic and aluminium, from the body. There is scientific evidence in support of the theory that children with autism suffer from metal toxicity; and that removing these toxins reduces autism symptoms. Although there has been controversy over whether mercury has contributed to the increase in the number of children diagnosed with autism, the growing evidence in this regard can't be ignored.

Dr McCandless encouraged us to reduce David's exposure to toxins. However, David's low nutritional status was a concern that is common in children with autism, and before we could start chelation we had to ensure that his stores of essential nutrients – such as zinc, magnesium and certain amino acids – were at satisfactory levels. As he was deficient in a number of the vital amino acids, Dr McCandless ordered a customised amino-acid formula for David.

We followed up the chelation with infusions of essential minerals, including zinc and magnesium, to restore these vital nutrients to his already compromised system. Chelation can strip the body indiscriminately of both good minerals and bad toxins, and so we struggled to keep David's essential nutrients in check.

We also tried to ensure that David's gut health was in satisfactory condition before starting chelation therapy. The reason for this is explained in a chelation paper published by the Autism Research Institute:

> *At least 50% of children with autism suffer from constipation and/or diarrhoea. 95% of autistic children have extremely high levels of E coli and often other bacteria that produce high levels of endotoxins. Yeast dysbiosis may also be a concern. Some detoxification treatments can cause or exacerbate bacteria/yeast dysbiosis, either directly or indirectly by providing food to them or by causing excretion of toxic metals into the gut.*
>
> (http://www.collegepharmacy.com/images/download/DAN_Chelation_Protocol_Position_Paper.pdf)

We thus had to be very sure that David's gut health was up to standard.

Cleaning up David's environment

A critical step was to reduce any toxic exposure in David's environment. If we were going to chelate him, we had to ensure that his world was clear of contaminants. One of the first steps in treating children with autism is securing a clean, non-toxic environment for them and reducing any toxic overload contributing to autism symptoms.

Shattered glass and shattered nerves

At the age of three David would often suffer from high fevers which would go on and on for days. Being a first-time mom, I'd take his temperature regularly. The reading would reach 40 degrees Celsius most times. David would be curled in a ball on the bed, eyes droopy and cheeks flaming red from fever. He'd start to shiver and this would cause his fever to climb even more. I'd sponge him down in an attempt to keep him cool and bring down his temperature. We'd dip a wet rag in room-temperature water, wring out the water and wipe his steaming forehead and body.

Night after night I'd be awake, sleeping next to him, as I nursed him through what felt like uncontrollable fevers that just wouldn't break. Even though sleep would overcome me in the early hours of the morning, I'd force myself awake to check on him.

We'd give him ibuprofen and sometimes Voltaren suppositories to bring down the raging fevers. He wouldn't be allowed paracetamol as this lowers GSH and ibuprofen doesn't. I used to worry that his fevers would cause convulsions.

Oral antibiotics were not an option for David and, although this was beyond scary, we fought the fevers without them. The days merged into one and I never knew which day of the week it was. Time stood still and I was stuck in David's world of fevers. It was physically and emotionally draining. I didn't eat for days, and was unable to remember the last time I had had food. I didn't have much of an appetite. Seeing him suffer through the fevers was heart-wrenching and worrisome. Many young, developing children fall ill, but David's fevers were relentless and would occur over and over again. Later on, I'd learn that this can be common in some children with autism.

During one bout of fever, I used the standard, traditional glass thermometer containing mercury to measure his temperature. I inserted it under his arm and counted down three minutes by my watch. I'd just taken the reading and was shaking the thermometer rigorously to get it back down to zero when the glass knocked the knuckles of my other hand and shattered the thermometer into tiny pieces onto the carpeted floor. The frightening part was that the silver mercury from the thermometer rolled into thousands of tiny balls across the room. As the mercury danced across my bedroom floor, I became hysterical and started crying and screaming. I was petrified as I knew that mercury exposure was dangerous for David.

My mother happened to be with me on that fateful day and she slapped me across the face in an attempt to calm me down.

I called Martin. I was frantic and hardly able to get the words out to explain what had happened. We'd been working so hard to clean up his environment I had no idea how I'd restore our bedroom to its previous mercury-free state. He sprang into action and we decided to replace the carpet just to be safe. Within an hour, a team of carpet installers knocked on my door and got to work replacing the damaged carpet with a brand new one. I sighed with a deep sense of relief when they left, thankful that the room had been restored to its previous mercury-free state. Apart from the smell of new carpet, all was forgotten by the time we crept into bed that night.

Three days later, David's fever was still raging unrelentingly. It never dawned on me to get him an electronic thermometer as I was too busy caring for him to think about leaving his side for a moment to go to the shops. I had a few old glass thermometers, and I was going to be sure to be very careful in order to prevent myself from smashing another one.

I was exhausted and worn down from David's fevers, not to mention the uneasiness which periodically crept into my mind over David's delayed development. I longed for him to speak, never daring to even dream about what his voice could or would sound like. I just couldn't imagine it. All therapies and educational interventions were put on hold during David's many rounds of high fever and sickness – which didn't help my state of mind when I knew that we were working against the clock every day. As the days passed by, my fear was that he was missing out on valuable instruction; and so we tried everything possible to restore his health.

What happened next sounds ridiculous and unbelievable, but I broke yet another glass thermometer and once again witnessed silver balls of mercury flying across our bedroom. To Martin's disbelief, utter shock and dismay, he fielded yet another call from his distressed wife rambling on about mercury spreading across the brand-new carpet in our bedroom. For a second time, the same team of carpet installers appeared at my door. I can only imagine how crazy they must have thought I was to be replacing a three-day-old carpet. Needless to say, we then bought an electronic thermometer.

Not knowing what to do about a terrifying fever

High temperatures are something nearly every parent goes through with their child at one time or another. But with David – as Ilana relates above – this was a great deal scarier.

When parents call doctors for advice on their child's high fever, the usual answer they receive is to give their child Panado or paracetamol. But David wasn't most children. When he had a high fever, we'd give him possibly the highest dose of paracetamol you could give and it simply didn't touch sides. When we told the paediatrician what we'd done he said to double the dose because 'you can't overdo paracetamol. It's very difficult to overdose on it.' So we doubled the dosage again – and it still didn't make any difference.

Now our child was burning up. We'd given him the highest dose possible and there was still no change. We were worried about convulsions, so now we called the paediatrician in panic. And, of course, you couldn't get through to him: you had to page him and get him to phone you. This could be hours later – sometimes you would have to call a second or third time.

By now you're waiting on the edge of your seat for this doctor to phone because your child is burning up and getting worse and worse. It's one thing to have a fever for one or two days, but after seven days he hasn't eaten and he's wasting away and you start to panic.

You eventually speak to the paediatrician who says there's nothing you can do – just sponge him down in a cool bath. This results in David screaming and crying because the water is tepid and uncomfortable, and we're still no closer to reducing the fever. If it came down slightly it would just as easily go back up again.

So after bathing didn't help we called our GP, who suggested Voltaren suppositories. We'd asked our paediatrician about Voltaren before and he had said definitely not – they're so bad for the child. They're dangerous. And his ultimate response when asked why we shouldn't give it? 'I just don't like it.'

By now, although we were petrified of giving Voltaren, we were desperate and thought, 'To hell with it, we can't carry on like this anymore.' So we gave David a Voltaren suppository and within an hour and a half the fever came plummeting down. If we'd had the courage to use it earlier (this was about our fifth bout of such fevers), we'd have saved ourselves so much heartache! With subsequent fevers, we could always rely on the Voltaren to work.

TESTING OUR DRINKING WATER

We tested our drinking water for parasites, metals, pesticides, lead, nitrate, coliform bacteria and anything else that could be harmful. You can get water contamination at almost any point in your delivery channel. Included here are lead leaking from corroded pipes, bacteria from cracked pipes and gardening chemicals. We inserted a reverse osmosis filter on our tap for David, and this worked well for us.

TESTING OUR BATH WATER

Even bath water can be a problem. We wanted to ensure that David bathed only in uncontaminated and clean water and installed a filter on the bath tap.

We also researched bath products, to make sure to avoid any chemicals that might be harmful to him.

TAKING A GOOD LOOK AT OUR SWIMMING POOL

One of David's greatest joys was splashing around in our pool. He could swim for hours on end, but we had noticed that as soon as he got out he would start 'ticking' (blinking his eye or developing a shoulder tick). We were horrified, and wondered if we had to add Tourette's syndrome to the never-ending list of David's problems.

We realised that David couldn't swim in a pool doused in chemicals and toxins and decided that the answer was a salt-water chlorinated pool. The problem is that you still have to add acid to this water in order to prevent green algae from growing. We soon learnt that acid caused David to have exactly the same reaction as with the other chemicals.

Next we investigated an ozone pool in the hope that it would solve our problem and allow David to swim. No luck – a lot of money later, and the result was the same.

The only place David can swim happily without any side effects is the ocean, which is why he so looks forward to holidays at the coast.

Trying out hyperbaric oxygen therapy

We made a point of keeping up to date with the latest developments on autism treatment and heard about hyperbaric oxygen therapy (HBOT) as a treatment. HBOT is defined as the medical use of oxygen at a higher than atmospheric pressure. The patient spends time in a special chamber that's pressurised in order to make more oxygen available to all body tissues.

Judy Chinitz was taking her son Alex for HBOT sessions in the United States, and we decided to research the possibility of finding a chamber in South Africa that could accommodate David. We called around checking whether hospitals in Johannesburg could provide HBOT. Initially, we had no luck finding a chamber that would allow me to go inside with David. By a stroke of good luck, however, we found a hard chamber in Boksburg that was exactly what we were looking for.

It wasn't going to be simple, though. The drive to the chamber would take me just under an hour one way. The whole exercise and round trip would take three hours a day. Determined to access the treatment against all odds, we nevertheless set the process in motion for HBOT. Driving on the highway to the chamber was gruelling and strenuous. There were many large trucks on this highway, and I felt very anxious driving there with David in the car.

Once we arrived at the chamber, it would take the HBOT operator ten minutes to get us up to pressure. During the dive down, I had to make sure that David was clearing his ears and equalising. I kept giving him sips to drink so he could unblock the building pressure in his ears. Once inside the chamber, we couldn't merely open the door if there was an emergency. If we wanted to use the toilet we'd have to wait at least ten minutes for the HBOT operator to bring us back up. It was daunting sitting in the chamber with David. It looked like a submarine and felt as if we were under the sea, trapped in a metal barrel with no escape.

From my seat in the chamber there was only a tiny round window giving me a sneak preview of the free world outside. No mobile phones or electronic devices were allowed in the chamber. My only means of communication with the outside world was an intercom which alerted the HBOT operator I needed assistance or that it was time to bring us back

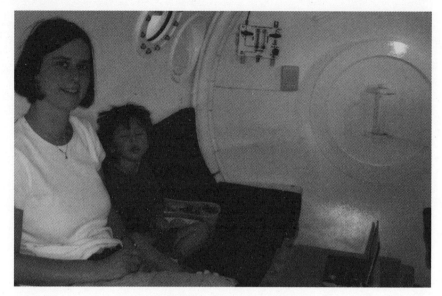

Ilana and David in the HBOT chamber

to the surface. Once we were in the chamber and at the right pressure, I'd place an oxygen mask over David's mouth. Initially it wasn't easy to secure the mask but in time David got used to it. It wasn't negotiable and I gave him no option but to get comfortable with the mask on his face.

Over time David became accustomed to the mask and the HBOT procedure. Time allows us to get used to almost anything, even though it would have been difficult for any four-year-old to sit in a chamber for an hour every day. David and I made the best of it and reconciled ourselves to the fact this was just something we did every day. The worst part was the loud noise of the machines operating the chamber. I can still hear the drone of the engine that sounded like an electric lawnmower. We had to bear the noise for an hour a day. However, this was a small price to pay considering the possible benefits of HBOT.

To say that it was a horrible experience is putting it mildly. From my window view I could see the barbed wire that outlined the HBOT centre's premises. I used to feel an overwhelming sense of sorrow when I stared at the barbed wire, as it reminded me that David and I were trapped in the world autism had created for us. I felt a deep sense of relief once the door opened and we were set free to travel home in the car. Although it took another hour to get home, at least I had control over my car and the journey back home and felt free and unencumbered.

But whatever it took, we were going to do everything possible to get David back. Some days I found myself juggling the IV infusions at the Charlotte Maxeke Hospital in the morning, followed by occupational and speech therapy, and finally HBOT in Boksburg.

THE RESULTS OF HBOT

Within a couple of weeks, we began to see an improvement in David's gut health. The oxygen he was getting from HBOT lowered the presence of anaerobic bacteria in his gut, decreased his inflammation and improved his immune function. HBOT also supported his detoxification, making him more alert and able to learn, and easier to manage behaviourally. There's no doubt David was better with the treatment than without – but sadly for him and us we were no closer in improving David's vocal, spontaneous and functional communication.

MARTIN'S TAKE ON HBOT

I learnt about HBOT on one of my trips to America and how it was benefiting kids with autism. Using a very sophisticated scanner, the studies showed that by using HBOT there was a lot more blood flow and brain activity in the language areas of the brain, and this resonated with us particularly.

For Ilana, battling through traffic to Boksburg and back was one thing but keeping David occupied in the chamber itself was another. David experienced what is called 'empty space' most of the time. If you didn't show him what to do or how to do it, he'd do absolutely nothing and simply stare into space. Kids generally *want* to play, even with a kitchen utensil if there's nothing else around. They don't always need fancy toys as they have imagination to occupy them. David, who had no imagination, was now in a chamber with nothing to occupy him for an hour at a time, not to mention the trial of trying to get him to keep his oxygen mask on and drink regularly. Clearing his ears was foreign to him, but we knew that if he didn't do it we could burst his eardrums going up or down in the chamber.

For the two of us, however, there was no mountain that was too high to climb to make even the smallest progress.

Managing nutrient supplementation

As if the diet wasn't enough to deal with, I had to manage David's nutrient-supplementation protocol. Soon after receiving that initial report from Dr McCandless, a big box of supplements from the United States arrived at our door.

Dr McCandless called children with autism 'children with starving brains'. Nutrient supplementation became an essential part of David's medical-treatment protocol. David's gut was inflamed and he suffered from gut dysbiosis and leaky gut. It made sense that he wasn't able to extract the vital nutrients and minerals he required for proper brain function from his food intake.

I remember slitting open the big brown box and packing out the bottles one by one. Like a kid in a candy store I pulled out one bottle after the next, placing them in the armoury of weapons I was collecting to treat David's autism. I never seemed to get to the bottom of the box. Vitamin supplements and minerals kept pouring out. The good news was that now we had extra ammunition to fight against autism. My kitchen cupboard was transformed into what looked like our very own home pharmacy.

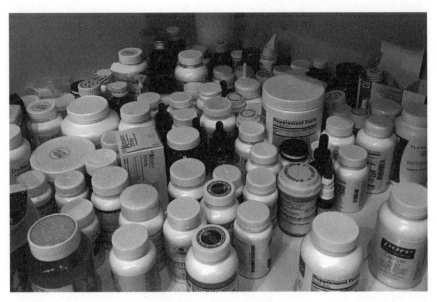

Our home pharmacy kitchen

Learning not to fear the label 'autism'

Parents and professionals are very often afraid of the word 'autism'. I used to be – until I became smarter than autism. When you're going to war, you need to know the enemy you're fighting against. For this reason, knowing your child has a diagnosis of autism is useful. Once your enemy is unmasked, you're in a position to plan your attack. We learnt early on that you don't win battles with a wooden spoon; and planned our strategy and armed ourselves with atomic weapons instead. Some treatments worked and others didn't help at all. When it wasn't working, we'd rethink our treatment plan and hold on to faith. We became creative and would plan a new strategy. Along the winding road we travelled, we learnt there are always solutions. It's never just the end of the road.

First realising that your child has autism is similar to being a wounded soldier on the battlefield. You find yourself lying face down on the ground injured, and there are bullets flying over your head. You try to take cover, but fear overcomes you and you stand frozen, unable to make a move. The choice is yours. You can lie there and succumb to your wounds or crawl wounded to the helicopter on the hill that will airlift you to safety. No one can assure you of making it home – but you do have a choice. Even though we were wounded, we chose to crawl as fast as we could to safety.

CLOSE YOUR EYES AND OPEN YOUR MOUTH

It was daunting to think that David would be required to swallow so many supplements in one day. I looked at the bottles in astonishment, wondering how I was going to get my two-year-old son to take all these supplements. There were capsules of different sizes, varying in colour and composition, and there was omega oil in liquid form that smelt very fishy and tasted ghastly. Certain supplements had to be taken half an hour before food and others half an hour after food. I memorised David's supplement regime off by heart, leaving no room for error.

David *had* to take the supplements and I'd find a way to get them down. If taking the supplements was important to his health and improved his functioning, I was going to make sure he swallowed every single one. Initially, I mixed the foul-smelling, bitter-tasting powders into a home-made pear sauce I steamed and blended. Later on, I found a better solution by warming pear sauce in the microwave. Placing a small amount of warm pear sauce on a teaspoon, I placed the capsule horizontally into the sauce. When I put the spoon in his mouth, he swallowed quickly because the sauce was hot. He soon learnt that when the spoon with pear sauce was placed in his mouth, he had to swallow. Years later, I'd learn that there are feeding experts who teach children how to swallow pills.

Sleep disturbance all round!

David struggled to fall asleep – and to stay asleep. Autism held us and our son hostage night after night, by never allowing David or us a peaceful night's sleep. We all became its victims.

David would wake up at 1 am or 2 am; and would remain awake for two or three hours at a time. We rocked him repetitively for hours and hours in the hope that he would fall asleep. Eventually, we rocked him so much that we broke the white wooden rocking chair in his room. We replaced the chair with his pram and wheeled him up and down the driveway for hours. Night after night, he'd wake from his sleep.

On the rare occasions when he didn't wake up, I'd lie awake waiting for him to wake up. If he did sleep through the night, he'd be awake by 5 am. Exhaustion set in for him and for us. We couldn't function without sleep and neither could David.

Sleep deprivation caused David and us much anguish and heartache. Martin and I were physically and emotionally drained. It became extremely taxing to stay calm and function properly. Taking the right decisions while being sleep-deprived can be challenging. Recognising this, we decided to take turns spending a weekend in a hotel to catch up on sleep. David's abnormal sleep pattern is a common problem for children with autism.

Overwhelming demands

The demands and expectations placed on us at the time felt overwhelming. Special diets, supplement protocols, blood draws, calls and visits to doctors and therapists, and learning about the dos and don'ts of autism all took a great deal of time and money. While juggling all this, we still had to work in order to pay the bills. And there was Eli, who also needed our time and attention. Raising children who are developing typically, without complications or the need for long lists of special requirements, *can* be taxing – but raising David was so much more demanding. On top of that, we didn't have the necessary support from friends or family, especially in the early days when we were still settling into the diagnosis and finding our feet.

Early on we learnt who our true friends really were; and as a result surrounded ourselves only with friends and family members who raised us up. There has been no time for negativity or trivial family spats since the diagnosis that changed all our lives.

CHAPTER SEVEN

FINDING DAVID'S VOICE

It was March 2007 and we were anxiously waiting for more test kits to arrive from the United States. Testing David's blood, urine and stool was required at regular intervals in order to direct treatment. Once the test kits finally arrived, we had to familiarise ourselves with how to do the sample collection. This involved drawing David's blood and sending the samples to the laboratories in Johannesburg. Sending samples to the United States required careful planning. The worst part was waiting for the US laboratories to analyse the samples and release the test results to Dr Bradstreet.

Next came a Skype consultation with Jeff to interpret the results, and then we had to organise with the US pharmacies to purchase and ship the items we needed for David's treatment. As there's a time difference between South Africa and the United States, we had to plan the calls, taking into account the seven-to-ten-hour time difference between our countries. Calling our credit card company to warn them to expect an international transaction and to keep the card open happened frequently and took time to arrange.

Overcoming distance
We had to consider customs and shipping details. Some pharmacies in the US can only ship to certain states within America and this proved challenging. We'd have to ask favours of people who knew someone who knew someone else who was coming to South Africa and could bring us the

medications.

Once the items had arrived at our door despite all the odds, we had to work out how to administer them. This all took time, which was something David didn't have on his side. *Early diagnosis and treatment are pivotal to recovery.* The window of opportunity stays open for only a very brief moment: by the time you stop to look back and take stock, years have passed and the window is closing.

In a desperate attempt to save David, we did everything possible to fast-track all the details involved in planning and following a medical-treatment regime. At the same time, of course, we continued to create and reinvent David's education and rehabilitation on a constant basis.

The deafening sound of silence

How I longed to hear my son's voice! This longing became a pain that was indescribable. Knowing he was incapable of communicating with us followed me around like a shadow. I was determined to find the key to unlock his voice. I developed a deep, unbearable desire to hear him speak. I was going crazy inside my head, heartbroken and tormented by the situation. I prayed and prayed and wept and prayed some more. I bargained with G-d to make me ill instead, or to take my life in return for David's voice.

I wanted him to tell me what he wanted to eat and which movie he wanted to watch on TV. I wondered about his favourite colour or if he loved me. How could we be robbed of hearing his sweet little voice commenting on the aeroplane that flew over or the dog barking in the park? Why this had happened to my child was a question I'd regularly ask myself, wondering how we were going to turn this around. Eli used to ask me why David couldn't speak. I explained to Eli that G-d had made him the 'talker boy' instead of David.

There has to be a way …

How can any parent be expected to accept that their child won't be able to communicate? It's unthinkable and unimaginable to suggest to any parent that their child will remain without communication for life. Had I been incorrectly led to believe that David would never speak and would remain incapable of this basic skill all his life? Surely, we'd find a way: after all, David was a human being and deserved a voice. It would be unjust to expect that David should be robbed of this basic human right – communication. There was no way I was going to stand by and let autism keep his voice locked away forever. There was a lot at stake and I wasn't prepared to lose.

Every breath I took was agonising in those early years, as all I could think and talk about was how I was going to get David to communicate. We clung desperately to every approximation of the sounds he tried to produce. The days turned to weeks and the weeks to months. As time flew by, David didn't make the progress we'd hoped and prayed for. I was overcome by fear and concern for his future and ours.

I bargained with autism in the early hours of the morning when I shook awake from sleep remembering the harsh reality that my child couldn't speak. Autism had hijacked David and held his voice hostage. Determined to free him, we planned and redesigned our strategy daily, checking in on the day's plan of action. I took a decision that I wasn't going to negotiate with his hostage taker; I was going to kill autism with one big blow to the head. I followed autism night and day like a hunter stalks its prey, waiting for the right moment to attack.

One day when my psychologist asked me how I was feeling, I replied that I had no feelings at all. I was not happy or sad, or even angry; and I felt nothing for a very long time. One day, after months of sessions with him, I saw his face light up. He told me to pick up the lighter next to my cigarette box on the table and said: 'Light it and put your finger in the flame.'

I did this and he asked, 'Did you feel that?' 'Yes!' I replied.

To him, that was a sign that my ability to sense my feelings had been restored. Confirmation came later that evening, when a friend came by to tell me about a car accident earlier that day in which both the driver and the passenger had died instantly. I heard myself saying, 'That makes me feel sad.' This was a breakthrough, as I'd had no normal feelings for years!

Discovering PROMPT

David was five years old. I woke up one morning and called Judy. I confided in her and conveyed my frustration about David's inability to communicate. She asked me if we had considered using a technique called PROMPT (Prompts for Restructuring Oral Muscular Phonetic Targets). When I put the phone down I ran to my computer, turned it on and googled PROMPT. The PROMPT Institute founded by Deborah Hayden in the United States popped up. I scanned the website, soaking up the information. I summoned Martin from work, causing him to run out of an important meeting so we could plan our PROMPT strategy.

David, like many other children with autism, had apraxia (a motor-speech challenge) and struggled to plan sounds and words at the motor level. PROMPT endeavours to teach the muscles involved in speech how to round and contract in order to produce the different sounds and words. The more we read about PROMPT, the more it made sense and the more I knew we had to use this tool with David.

Children with autism suffer from brain inflammation, which breaks the synapses (wiring) in the brain, causing an interruption in signalling from the brain to the facial muscles responsible for speech. In an attempt to bridge this interruption in signalling, PROMPT uses tactile cues to the facial muscles to assist a child in overcoming apraxia. PROMPT is a game changer.

Bringing PROMPT to South Africa

On the same night I discovered PROMPT, I rang Deborah Hayden in the United States. After a couple of my attempts to reach her, she eventually picked up the phone. I initially froze when I heard her voice on the other end of the line, wondering what I was going to say to her. I explained that we lived in South Africa and that I'd researched her website and wanted to learn about how PROMPT could help David's apraxia. I invited her to come to South Africa as she could go on safari as well as run training in PROMPT. The word 'safari' sealed the deal.

Throughout our journey, we managed to find a way to access people at the top of their organisations. We didn't speak to assistants, and instead made sure to speak directly to the top person. I suspect that being a South African and far away had a lot to do with our success in reaching these experts. Had I been a local American, I would have just been referred to the local PROMPT therapist in my state. Directly reaching Deborah, the founder and CEO of the PROMPT Institute, was a real win.

I was disappointed, though, when I learnt that she could only come to South Africa six months later. I wasn't willing to wait six months and therefore Deborah suggested that we first make a trip to Austin, Texas, to consult with her senior partner. She undertook to book a trip to South Africa but made an interim arrangement for me to visit Texas. The plan was to teach me how to continue with PROMPT once I returned home with David.

The Texan challenge

One week after speaking to Deborah, David and I boarded a plane and set off on the long trip to Austin, Texas, which is a daunting one with any five-and-a-half-year-old, let alone one with autism. I packed a large bag of gadgets, changes of clothes, and food David liked. It was unnerving to think how I was going to keep him occupied on the long flight to New York, and from there to Austin. I packed kosher gluten- and dairy-free foods for the trip. It wasn't as if we could eat the airline food or enjoy the excitement of it! We were adhering to David's diet as strictly as ever.

We said goodbye to Martin and went through to catch our flight. As I moved towards the plane with David, I choked back the tears and bravely braced myself for the long trip ahead. By the time I had walked onto the plane, however, I was sobbing quietly. I wiped away the tears with the back of my hand, holding David's hand and the big heavy black bag with all our stuff in it and walked down the aisle to our seats. I was petrified for so many reasons. I hardly ate or drank anything for days.

We arrived in New York after an 18-hour flight and stood for two hours in a queue for passport control that wound around the arrival terminal. I was constantly aware that David could have a serious meltdown any minute and create a massive scene. After a long flight I didn't know how much more waiting David could handle.

Once I got through passport control I had to manage David and the bags on my own. I flagged down a yellow cab to take us to the hotel. When we arrived I went up to the room with David, oblivious of the fact I'd forgotten to change the time on my watch. There was a swimming pool in the hotel and as David enjoyed swimming I took him down to the pool to paddle around before we were picked up to go to Judy's house. The plan was to spend time with Judy and Dr Alan Greenstein, a well-known autism doctor, and then catch an early 6 am flight to Austin the next morning.

David was swimming around in the pool when a hotel attendant came to call me. My pick-up had arrived to take me to Judy's house and was waiting outside. My heart skipped a beat and I realised I was two hours behind schedule. I was about to fly out of the pool to get dressed when I noticed two long brown logs submerged under the water. I knew instantly that David had produced these. I stood there in shock for at least 30 seconds, contemplating my options. I'm ashamed to say I pulled David out of the water and made a run for it ...

Meeting Judy

It was a 45-minute drive to Judy's house. As we sat in the car my phone rang unexpectedly. Surprised to hear Dr Rodney's voice on the other end of the line, I asked him if everything was okay as I wondered why he was calling me at around 2 am South African time. He said: 'Ilana, listen carefully to me. You can consult with doctors and therapists, but you must also find the spiritual channel that will lead to David's full recovery. I've arranged for a pick-up for you and David at 9 pm New York time. You'll be taken to the grave of the Lubavitcher Rebbe (the Rebbe is considered one of the most influential Jewish leaders of the 20th century). It's a spiritual site and it's customary to pray at the gravesite. I'm not taking no for an answer so make sure you're ready at 9 pm.' I thanked him and put the phone down. We were exhausted and I had no idea how I would manage the outing he'd arranged. In my heart, however, I knew it was important. I trusted Dr Rodney, and so I went along with what he'd scheduled for us.

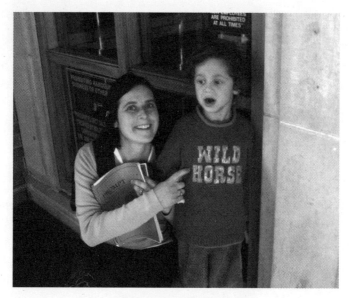

A trip to PROMPT, in Texas

Judy had been a guiding light to us for many years and meeting her was really emotional for me. She taught us about autism treatment and walked beside us, holding us up on our journey. Judy spent every waking moment looking for a cure for autism. She has been instrumental in helping many children find their way home from autism. We spent time with her and Dr Greenstein, discussing David's treatment plan. Time passed quickly and we had to say goodbye.

Spiritual upliftment

By the time we arrived at the Rebbe's gravesite, David had fallen asleep. I lay him down next to the grave as I held the prayer book in my hand, my lips reciting the *Psalms*, my heart pouring out my emotions and prayers. I prayed for his speedy and full recovery, begging for mercy and an end to our suffering. As the tears rolled down my face and dropped beneath me to the ground, I prayed for strength and for David to be healed.

It was late at night and as we turned to go, leaving behind the cemetery, I felt an enormous sense of peace in my heart. I knew I'd done everything possible to secure and pave the way home for David. I was fighting this war on both a physical and a spiritual level, and that had to lead to victory.

I'd learn years later that suffering isn't always a punishment; and can simply be a test of faith. A false perception is that life should be a journey in a luxury car with air conditioning, along a smooth and picturesque tar road, while we sit on the backseat sipping an ice-cold drink. For us, life became a walk in the hot sun along a gravel road that wasn't picturesque or smooth. We walked barefoot on the long, hot road with no shoes to protect the soles of our feet. We had no choice but to put one foot in front of the other, ignore the pain, the heat of the sun and our overwhelming thirst. We just had to keep walking.

BOARDING THE PLANE TO AUSTIN

I was woken by my alarm at 4 am. I had to get our bags packed for our 5-am pick-up to catch the flight. I was exhausted and forced myself to wake up and get everything ready.

At the airport I was dumped unceremoniously on the side of the road with two big suitcases, numerous bags and David clinging to me. As I watched the taxi drive off, I stood there wondering how I'd move us and our luggage inside the terminal. I managed to do what felt like an impossible task and we boarded the plane to Austin. When we landed, there was no one to greet us or offer us a lift to the hotel. We were hungry and food became quite a challenge, considering David's diet and my vegetarian kosher requirements.

After checking in to the hotel we took a shuttle to a store called Wholefoods. Experiencing Wholefoods was utterly mind-blowing. I'd never imagined there could be such a variety of good, wholesome and delicious-tasting food available to people who needed a special diet. From gluten-free to dairy-free to yeast-free, you name it, they had it. The almond milk and YumEarth lollipops were particularly exciting finds. I loaded my trolley with organic lollipops of all flavours for David. I felt like I was in heaven. We spent two hours at Wholefoods, walking up and down the aisles and piling our trolley with colourful treasures of legal goodies for David.

Learning PROMPT

I spent two gruelling weeks with David in Austin learning the PROMPT technique. In the morning we'd spend time with the PROMPT instructor; and in the afternoon we consulted with an expert in ABA, based at the Center for Autism and Related Disorders office in Austin.

PROMPT was everything I'd hoped it would be. I was elated and confident we'd found a solution. The physical, tactile prompts to the face made sense to me. PROMPT wasn't offered by any South African speech therapist and had never been mentioned to me as a treatment option. In fact, I'd been told I could equate David's condition to that of a child in a wheelchair who had severed their spine and couldn't walk. In the same way, David wouldn't talk. When the speech therapist told me on that fateful day that David would *never speak*, I told myself: 'She just said he may speak.' I *never* took no for an answer. I'd followed my gut and was relieved to see I'd taken the right decision bringing David to Austin. Here we were, learning a brand-new method to help David speak. I was super excited.

The PROMPT instructor started the treatment by conducting an assessment of David's motor-speech hierarchy. The aims of this assessment were to evaluate David's motor-speech system and to identify the level or stage at which his problems were occurring. The assessment would also give us information on which motor domains required attention.

The assessment revealed a number of specific deficits. Firstly, David's phonatory control was inadequate, meaning that his ability to control and sustain his breath was not good enough for speech. He would have trouble turning his voice off to make sounds like *p*, *t*, and *h*, and he'd have trouble turning his voice on for sounds like *b*, *d* and *ah*. He also couldn't sustain his breath long enough to produce a word like *mom* or *dad*, and he couldn't turn his voice on and off within a word like *hat* or *sit*.

Secondly, his mandibular control was weak. Most people talk within four jaw heights, the smallest being used for a sound like *m*, and the biggest for a sound like *ah*. Most people with good mandibular control don't open their jaws wider than necessary to insert two of their fingers between their top and bottom teeth. David's jaw was almost slack, and he'd make very large movements with his jaw, making it hard for him to produce any of the many small-jaw sounds.

Thirdly, David's labial-facial control was poor. He had trouble retracting (pulling back) his lips for sounds like *ee* or *s*, and he didn't round his lips neatly for sounds like *oo* or *oh*.

The assessment was unable to target the areas of sequenced movement (being able to connect sounds in words, phrases and sentences) because this was too high-level in relation to David's development at that stage. There was no point to trying to work at the word or sentence level when the sound level was not in place.

Prosody too was not a short- or medium-term goal at the time, because it is concerned with things such as intonation. Again, we needed to help him produce sounds clearly and start forming words before worrying about that aspect of things.

The trainer was hopeful that, with a PROMPT plan designed specifically for him, David would be able to make the necessary changes over time, and that these would ultimately result in his being able to use his voice.

The next step was the design of David's own PROMPT programme. I had come prepared and pulled out my video recorder to tape the delivery of the prompts, so I could capture on tape exactly how the PROMPT instructor manipulated David's facial muscles.

PROMPT is a tactile-kinaesthetic approach that addresses the development of sensory-motor processing. The method involves touch, pressure and targeted placements on the face. Through complex tactile touches to the face, prompting each muscle responsible for a specific sound, the instructor guided David into producing different sounds.

OVERCOMING AN UNEXPECTED ROADBLOCK

I was told I wouldn't be able to videotape PROMPT as it was the PROMPT Institute's rule not to allow video recording. This couldn't be right. I'd flown halfway across the world to learn this technique, only to be told I wasn't allowed to catch the prompts on camera! I insisted on the recording, wresting permission from the PROMPT instructor, and made the recording. Emotionally and physically sapped by it all, I recorded with shaking hands as the instructor showed me how and where to touch the facial muscles to manipulate speech and create new neuro-motor maps for speech.

David's Pica and the Center for Autism and Related Disorders

Our main goal in flying to Austin had been for me to learn PROMPT. The PROMPT Institute would only see us and train me in PROMPT for two hours a day, which left the rest of the day open with not much to do. I decided to make contact with the Center for Autism and Related Disorders (CARD). To my amazement, the CARD office was in the same road as the PROMPT Institute. I could only gain from visiting them, to learn as much as I could to help David.

CARD offered what they called out-patient services for specific maladaptive behaviours. David's Pica, an eating disorder that involves eating a variety of non-food items such as sand or paper and is common in children with autism, was out of control. One of their doctors was enrolled to do what they called a 'functional analysis' on David's Pica to determine its cause and the best course of action to prevent it from reoccurring.

Pica can stem from nutritional deficiency and we first had to do tests to rule this out. We'd screened David for these deficiencies before, but his Pica continued irrespective of all the nutrient supplementation we gave him. I learnt that it was possible for Pica to extend beyond the correction of its medical cause – it could become a 'learnt behaviour' (an incorrect behaviour you have the desire to do over and over again because it makes you feel good), serving a specific function for the child.

The truth is that, as much as David's Pica was an issue, I wanted contact with CARD to determine if they could be of use to David and me in any way. The doctor directing the functional analysis took David and me to a room where she had placed non-edible items on the floor to test his Pica. We left David in the room and watched through a glass window, gathering data on the frequency with which he'd engage in eating the non-edible items scattered around the room.

We needed to take the data over a couple of days to get accurate statistics on the frequency and reasons for David's Pica. The purpose of the functional analysis was to determine the function of the behaviour. Was David's Pica automatic, or did he engage in this behaviour for the purpose of attention, to escape from tasks, or for any other reason?

ABA again provides an answer

As the time went by, the CARD doctor and I forged a bond. When she handed me the report on the last day, she had concluded that David's Pica was automatic. She asked me to remain in Austin to conduct a colonoscopy for David, as she suspected he had severe bowel inflammation. I felt so helpless listening to her, as this was nothing new to us and we had been doing all we could to change the problem for such a long time …

The doctor also told me that, even though David was five years old, we should consider ABA treatment for him and that it wasn't too late for him to develop speech even though he would require many hours of ABA. She was sad to see us go and told me that she wouldn't allow me to board the plane home to South Africa. David had crawled into her heart. She wanted me to stay in Austin so she could help us with David's ABA programme. Even though staying wasn't an option, it felt good to be supported and to have it confirmed that more could be done. This gave me hope when I really needed the boost.

I promised her we'd consider ABA once I returned home. I did make contact with the CARD Austin office, but the cost of bringing ABA to South Africa seemed exorbitant at the time. This was a big mistake, one we would regret years later.

Bringing PROMPT to South Africa

Deborah Hayden arrived in South Africa six months after my trip to Austin and we showed her around Johannesburg. I co-ordinated her schedule and arranged for the first training of speech therapists in South Africa in the PROMPT technique. This was groundbreaking for the speech therapy profession in South Africa. In the years to follow, we trained many more speech therapists in PROMPT, entrenching the technique on the continent.

CHAPTER EIGHT

THE BIRTH OF LITTLE STARS

Once I arrived back in Johannesburg armed with the knowledge and videos on PROMPT I'd taken in Austin, I was determined to use this technique to get David to talk. At that time it was me alone, with no support structure or staff on what is a very technical, time-consuming method. It's also never a good idea to be both mom and instructor.

I'd regularly send Deborah short video clips of me working with David using PROMPT. She'd send me feedback that basically tore my work to shreds. I started wondering whether in fact I was doing more harm than good. It was incredibly frustrating: I knew I'd found a key to unlocking David's voice, but the challenge was delivering it in the right way. I did the best I could, but David's gains were not measurable enough.

Searching for a school

Later on that year, I visited various special-needs schools. What I saw was simply horrific and I'd return home in tears, taken aback by the horrendous state of affairs I experienced during my explorations. I couldn't understand how children with different diagnoses, ages and abilities could be grouped together in one class with one teacher and one facilitator. What I observed, instead of expert schools catering for the needs of their learners, were care facilities lacking expertise, funding, equipment and staff.

Autistic children were grouped together with physically disabled children – with neither group's needs being met. I visited one school after another, and what I saw was concerning. One of the schools tied the children to their chairs in an attempt to get them to pay attention. I couldn't find a single special-needs school that impressed me with its credentials or staff training. The facilities we visited, in my opinion, were merely babysitting the children.

I spent time at a school that had a so-called 'good reputation' for autism and we attended a class consisting of ten children with varying diagnoses and learning challenges. The teacher assisted one of the children who couldn't walk or talk to colour in a page on the desk in front of her, forcing her to complete the task. Her desperate screams for help resonated throughout the room as she protested. She didn't look down at the page, not even once, and I felt physically ill watching the scene unfold before us.

The child became so distressed that she fell on the floor and had a seizure. During this time, I wondered who was giving the other nine challenged children the individualised attention *they* needed. It was clear to me this class set up wasn't going to work for me and David. Once the child came around, it was break and the assistant carried her to the old broken rusted jungle gym outside in the garden. I asked the teacher where the playground was and she indicated that we were standing in it. It was alarming to me that this facility was so poorly staffed and run down.

I said my goodbyes and left with David, knowing there was no way I'd dump him somewhere – just so I could have free time away from him and carry on my life with no expectations or hopes of him reaching his potential. I wondered how any parent could send their child to the school I'd just seen. The only reason I could think of was that parents become desperate and eventually succumb to the dismal options available to them. Teachers who lack experience, knowledge and teaching skills mislead parents into believing they should accept their child's fate and not set any expectations for the children. Their experience is very narrow and they lack expert training. The parents then become convinced that there's no better facility for their child; and that they need to accept their 'disabled' child as sadly limited.

I wasn't going to accept that my child was destined to be dumped at some inadequate facility, forgotten and written off by the school system. The only thing I accepted was that I needed to work harder to find the right educational programme for my son. I was determined to ensure he'd be placed in professional hands. David deserved a future – and I was going to do everything possible to turn the world upside down to find what I was looking for to secure his education.

Surely, my son deserved the best teachers, equipment and support staff to give him the education he so desperately required to help him function as a human being. I soon realised that the school I envisaged just didn't exist. It was an upsetting experience to travel around from one special-needs school to the next, and I held out little hope I'd find what I was looking for in my quest to enrol David in a quality school.

The bitter end

I visited another Johannesburg school, one highly recommended for autistic children. Upon my arrival, I was taken to meet the principal, whose ideals and vision for autistic children I didn't share. Her lack of knowledge on the causes and treatments of autism concerned me and I couldn't leave my son's education and future in the hands of someone who wasn't an expert and who hadn't kept up with the latest developments. I watched children aimlessly walking around during break, and I left the school disturbed, knowing instinctively this wasn't the right placement for David.

A long list of private schools catering for the educational needs of typically-developing children and offering luxury facilities and only the best-trained teachers was available to the parents of 'normal' children. These parents could select the school that best suited their child's needs. The focus was on excellence and achievement. It felt to me that no one cared about children with a difference – children who truly needed the best facilities to secure their future.

I finally decided to visit one of the mainstream schools in our area, to ask if they'd consider accepting David along with a facilitator, and the response I got was that the parents of the other children were not ready for a child with autism. It would be disturbing for the parents and the learners to be exposed to autism, and therefore they couldn't consider my request. Years later, I would question the legality of this decision.

How could a school that claimed to teach their children good morals and values turn us away, based on the fact that the parents and children were not ready to experience autism? Surely all children should be exposed to difference and given the opportunity to experience the challenges of others less fortunate than themselves? This would inevitably create a great learning opportunity for the more 'typical' learners. We were rejected and sent away without consideration or a second thought.

Today, the inclusion of children like David in mainstream education has become more widely accepted around the world – but sadly not yet in South Africa.

My 'aha' moment

Martin refused to believe the ideal school didn't exist and encouraged me to keep looking.

It was now December 2007, and we were on a break at the coast. David's time was running out. He'd be turning six soon. It felt as if we were losing the battle against autism. His progress was too slow.

Martin and I discussed our options. We knew we were in trouble. Our hopes and dreams of a bright future for David were slowly slipping away. We needed to do something drastic and fast.

I screamed at the universe in the hope I'd receive a sign or message to guide us. I was standing on the balcony of our holiday apartment looking at the sea churning when the answer came to me: Everything we needed right then was in the United States!

Whether or not to emigrate from South Africa

We weighed up the pros and cons, and took a definitive decision to immigrate to the States. We hadn't just arrived at our decision. A gradual order of events had led us there, starting with a hunt for a school for David. We'd become frustrated with the lack of expert educational facilities for David; and trying to access the medical treatments and PROMPT support had begun to take its toll on us.

We researched schools for David in the United States and found one in New Jersey that appealed to us. Martin would remain in South Africa for the first year while I moved to the States and, over time, would transition there. I remember feeling heartbroken that our family would be torn apart by autism.

'We're staying'

Our decision to move to America consumed us. Martin was busy planning how he'd break the news that we'd be emigrating to his partner Bernie, who was also on holiday in Umhlanga. He'd been working with Bernie for ten years, and they shared the same ideals and had the perfect partnership. I'd felt sick over the previous two days, mulling over the details and plans we were making to move to America.

Martin went for a run with Bernie and along the way took a break on a bench next to the road. Once they were sitting down, he broke the news. But Bernie wasn't going to let Martin go easily – and came up with a long list of reasons why our move to the States might not be the answer. He told Martin we'd be in a new country learning a new system; and that this would take time away from our focus on David and his needs. We'd have to uproot our lives and split up our family. Bernie suggested we import what we needed from America and encouraged Martin to stay, offering his support to make this a reality. Little did Bernie know how his input would change the lives of so many other families like ours in South Africa …

Martin barged through the door after his run with Bernie, looked me in the eye and said: 'Change of plans – we're going to stay in South Africa and we'll import what we need for David'. An overwhelming sense of relief enveloped me, as I'd been very nervous and worried about emigrating with so much uncertainty and sacrifice required to make the move to the States.

Finding a home for Little Stars

We now took the decision to establish our own school; and, before we arrived home from our break, had already called estate agents to start looking for a property to match our specifications. On the first day back, we were taken around to view properties. The first property we walked into was a house in Highlands North. It was in the perfect area, with the ideal layout, and was sunny and bright. We had a good feeling about it and Bernie signed the offer to purchase. And so we became the proud beneficiaries of premises that would become the school we had dreamed about for David, with the best equipment and proficient staff, and filled with the energy and positivity we needed to secure our son's future.

We deliberated for days over a name for the school, and decided on Little Stars. We wanted to choose a name that would honour David. Little Stars seemed fitting as the Star of David, also known as the Shield of David, was a meaningful symbol and we felt pleased with our decision. The school would also be there to help autistic children reach for the stars.

Little Stars: a reality

We head-hunted an experienced speech therapist and special-needs teacher who had received her training in the UK at a prestigious school for autism, appointed her as our head teacher and briefed her on our vision for the school. She was experienced and passionate about working with children with autism, and we believed she would be able to deliver the educational programmes required.

I'd made friends with a mom whose son Daniel also had autism and went to the same occupational therapist as David. I called her excitedly to let her know we were establishing a school that would cater for the needs of autistic children; and that we would be importing the best teaching methodologies and strategies to ensure these children's success. Our school would be one of excellence, whose mission would be the advancement of children with autism. The focus would be on helping each child to catch up on their education; and on teaching them those skills they lacked but needed to make further progress.

We did some research and decided on four children, one teacher and two teaching aides per class, whom we'd train in the latest teaching methodologies for autistic children. We ordered only the best equipment and I was soon very busy managing the installation of a top-of-the-range jungle gym, trampoline and swings, and everything else we needed for the school. I ordered brand-new Occupational Therapy (OT) equipment and set up an OT room that offered the latest and best. If we couldn't find anything we needed locally, we ordered it from the United States and had it shipped to South Africa.

We advertised and interviewed a number of occupational therapists before selecting the most suitable candidate for Little Stars. We ordered new desks and chairs, and painted the school in pastel colours to create a warm, inviting environment to encourage learning. After a visit to the school, Daniel's mom was so impressed with my vision and what we had to offer that she happily enrolled her son at Little Stars.

We opened our doors and David and Daniel were the first students at the school. When I dropped off David every morning, I left confident and with the peace of mind that he was in the hands of a capable and professional team. I drew a certain amount of comfort from this knowledge and held out hope for his future.

Soon word of mouth spread and my phone started ringing with parents who'd heard about my school and wanted to enrol their children there. In a short space of time, we'd grown to 20 children and a long waiting list.

CHAPTER NINE

THE CHALLENGING CHILDREN CONFERENCE, JULY 2009

Taking stock

I had wrestled with autism day and night, trying to eradicate it from our lives. This remained a constant battle. Always on the look-out for new ways to tackle autism, I'd often need to re-evaluate David's treatment plan. This was physically and emotionally draining. I asked myself hard questions, having long discussions with Martin about whether the current plan was in fact yielding results. It would have been much easier to remain in a mindset where I'd convinced myself that David was doing well, when in fact this was not the case. I didn't allow doubt to stay hidden, safely tucked away in my subconscious – but rather confronted my thoughts and feelings. I no longer let fear rule me.

It was brave of us to admit to ourselves that our current strategy wasn't working, especially after we'd spent so much time, effort and money setting it up and rolling it out.

Not allowing autism to throw me off course

When I was a little girl my father bought me a Shetland pony as a birthday gift. I was so excited to take a ride on my pony, expecting the horse to trot across the field. Instead the pony was fierce and wild. I climbed on and as soon as I was secure in the saddle it ran straight for the barbed-wire fence of the enclosure. I was holding on for dear life, and wondering how the ride would end because the pony was ignoring my desperate tugs on the reins to slow it down. As the fence came closer I realised the pony was going to throw me onto the barbed wire. For a while I felt totally out of control – a terrible experience.

As we arrived at the fence, the pony predictably launched me into the air and onto the barbed wire. Once I had fallen beneath it on the ground, it continued to buck and kick its legs in the air. I didn't lie there long, however, even though I was in pain and had blood gushing from my arm. I decided to get up and climb straight back onto that horse. This time my expectations of the pony ride were different and the minute I got back in the saddle I took control – of the reins and the pony. That physical experience lay the foundation for how I would deal with autism later in my life. If autism threw me off course, I simply recalculated and got back on track.

I had to face the harsh reality that although David had made gains at Little Stars, I wasn't sufficiently happy with the outcome. After all the hard work, effort, financial outlay and time I'd poured into the project, David's progress never quite measured up to my expectations. While other children at Little Stars were doing well and their parents were happy, I became increasingly unsettled over time.

We were still consulting regularly with Dr Jeff Bradstreet, who always managed to rescue David from episodes of illness and kept our hope alive. I just couldn't believe there was no doctor in South Africa with the knowledge and experience to manage David in the same way as Jeff did.

There were many days when I felt sick with worry. Although I was alive, I wasn't present in this world. All I could talk about, think about, speak about and dream about was getting David to talk.

Changing the destiny of autism treatment in South Africa

During one of my moments of sadness, a thought entered my mind. If I could educate doctors in South Africa on the biomedical treatment protocol, the children at Little Stars could do even better. I didn't delay and emailed Jeff, offering him a ticket to South Africa and an invitation to present on biomedical treatments.

He replied almost immediately, accepting my invitation, and we set a time to discuss the details of his trip. What unfolded next would set the platform for reform in South Africa, changing the archaic notion that recovery from autism was impossible.

No doctor had presented on biomedical treatment in South Africa. Medical treatment that focused on identifying, targeting and addressing the underlying causes of autism wasn't spoken about or considered an option. It didn't exist. The prevailing view was that some children were simply autistic and required psychiatric medication to calm them down. Professionals were sometimes even reluctant to provide a diagnosis of autism because in their minds there really was no coming back from autism. During their studies they'd learnt that autism was a life-long disability and neurological condition – full stop.

Current research has shown that autism is epigenetic. This means that some children have a genetic vulnerability to developing autism. Should there be an environmental toxin or other trigger present, this may cause the gene responsible for the disease to 'express' itself.

I was determined to bring South Africa up to speed with the latest developments in autism treatment. I wanted to share everything Martin and I had learnt over the past seven years while flying to conferences in the United States and consulting with Jeff. If I could help other children get better, that might be the answer to helping David get better. I had nothing to lose.

Our next call with Jeff was one I often thought about later, as it was a defining moment that would end up affecting many lives. Jeff suggested that he bring Dr Doreen Granpeesheh, the founding director of CARD, with him to present on ABA.

My initial response was that we'd already tried ABA for David and it hadn't worked. What could Doreen possibly tell me that I didn't already know?

'What!' he exclaimed. 'Do you have any idea who she is? She's a leading world expert on autism and if you get the privilege of speaking to her you can consider yourself fortunate. She's extremely busy and is *the* authority on ABA and autism in America. You don't get to speak to the likes of

Doreen Granpeesheh. There's nothing to think about. CARD ABA is the best ABA in the world and you'd be foolish to turn down an opportunity to have her come to SA.'

He told me to think about it and let him know by morning. 'Doreen has a full schedule and I'd need to let her know soon so she can squeeze in the trip,' he added.

After the call, Martin and I sat outside on the couch, mulling it over. We couldn't disappoint Jeff. If he recommended her, she had to be good at what she did. It would mean an extra air ticket and more expense, but we took the decision that she should join Jeff. Once our decision had been made I immediately emailed him, confirming that Doreen should come too. It was the best decision we ever made and the next couple of months were filled with preparations for their trip.

Planning the conference

I knew nothing about co-ordinating an event. I sat down at my desk late one Saturday evening to get the ball rolling, suddenly realising that the first step had to be to name the conference I was planning. I considered whether professionals and parents might be put off by the word 'autism' and decided to call it the 'Challenging Children Conference' (CCC). If parents were in doubt as to whether their child in fact had autism, they'd relate to the word 'challenging' and this would convince them to attend. I didn't realise it then, but the work I put in over the next couple of months would be of fundamental importance to the future treatment of autism in Africa.

Every day for eight months I woke up and, after getting the kids dressed, fed and settled, I got to work making all the arrangements for the CCC. I had a logo designed and put together my first draft invitation. The next step would be to get the conference accredited through the Health Professions Council of South Africa, in order to secure continuing education units for the health professionals attending. This required an enormous amount of effort and paperwork but I got it done. I decided to arrange a separate doctors' lunch and Q & A for doctors, and invited a long list of general practitioners to attend free of charge.

I deliberated about approaching the media to interview Doreen and Jeff. I couldn't allow the world's leading experts on autism to come to South Africa without ensuring we reached as many people as possible with their important message – which was that autism is treatable.

Every day I'd call schools, inviting teachers to the conference. I sent the invitation to autism organisations, speech therapists, occupational therapists, psychologists and doctors and did my best to reach as many parents as possible, encouraging them to attend the upcoming event. I had long calls with parents who were asking for more information about the speakers and the topics to be covered. I took time to explain to everyone what information they'd receive at the conference.

Excitement builds

Very soon, the bookings started pouring in. I'd chosen a venue to seat 100 people but within the first three weeks of advertising I'd exceeded this figure and had to book the Linder Auditorium, which could seat 500 people. I set a new target for attendance and worked on spreading the word that the Conference would provide the latest cutting-edge and most up-to-date information on autism treatment.

From registration to hand-outs, organising the food and drinks, making the parking arrangements and hiring equipment, including a projector and microphone, I did it all on my own. I had no admin, office, personal assistant or events co-ordinator. The night before the conference when I tallied the attendees, I saw we had around 500 people attending. I emailed the list of attendees with the agenda for both days and made all the final arrangements.

I'd arranged a professional registration company to assist me. Each attendee received a name tag with their designation and the CCC logo. The professionals needed to receive certificates of attendance after the conference and I designed these and had them printed.

A few weeks before our keynote speakers arrived in South Africa, I received a call from the producer of a TV show called *Great Expectations*.

The show was presented by the well-known radio and TV personality Sam Cowan. The producer had received my email and was calling to ask if Ms Cowan could host Dr Bradstreet and Doreen live on air on the morning of their arrival. This was exhilarating news. When the producer suggested that Martin and I join them on set to share our experience of raising a child with autism, I froze, then heard myself agreeing to appear on the show. When I shared this idea with Martin he wasn't very keen, but he nevertheless agreed to join the panel. Maybe it was my stern stare that did it, but he realised we couldn't turn down the opportunity to be on TV.

I planned all the details on my list for Doreen and Jeff. I filled the vases in the house they were staying in with proteas and made dinner reservations at the finest African restaurant in town. I planned trips to the Lion Park and Nelson Mandela Square. They'd be going on safari during their stay in South Africa and I wanted them to have an unforgettable African experience.

Meeting Dr Jeff Bradstreet

The big day finally arrived. At 5 pm on the dot, the exact time his plane landed, we already stood in the arrivals hall anticipating the moment Jeff Bradstreet would walk through the doors. I could hardly breathe standing next to Martin waiting for him to arrive – I was so excited. Suddenly I looked up and there he was.

Once we'd checked Jeff into his accommodation, we sat around a table catching up and chatted to him like old friends meeting for a casual dinner date. I had to pinch myself because I couldn't believe we were finally meeting *the* authority on autism. We stayed chatting for hours and eventually said our goodbyes as Martin had to wake up early the next morning to meet Doreen at the airport. She was landing at 5 am and the plan was to drop her bags off at the residence and go straight to the TV studio.

Dr Doreen Granpeesheh

I felt very nervous about meeting Doreen. I'd done my research and knew

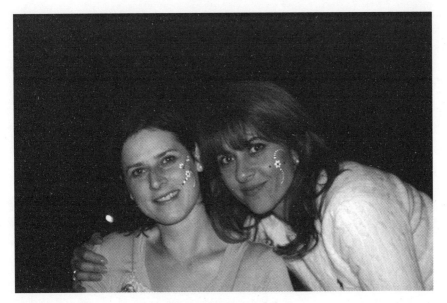

Dr Doreen Granpeesheh

she was more than just a well-respected autism authority. Yet the moment we met, she immediately crouched down in front of Eli so that she could be on the same level as he was. The interaction that followed between them spoke a thousand words. I stood watching them, and in that moment I knew she was kind and caring. Her natural empathy for children was evident and within a few minutes of meeting her I was surprised at how humble and warm she was.

Great expectations

We made our way to the TV studio in Hyde Park. Doreen drove with me and we spent time getting to know each other. The producer gave us a tour of the studios and briefed us on the logistics involved. The producer suggested that we avoid a discussion on vaccinations and their connection to autism, as she felt this might be a controversial topic not suitable for the show. We agreed and assured her we'd stay on topic.

We had our make-up and hair done and it was time to go on air. We entered the set and microphones were clipped to our lapels. Sam Cowan was sitting on a green couch waiting to interview us. There were sound technicians and studio assistants, taking care of all the details around us. There were cameras and bright lights, and for a brief moment I considered turning around and running out the door. I was shaking like a leaf. I hadn't slept at all the night before and was especially nervous.

The interview begins

Dr Bradstreet and Doreen were interviewed first.

Sam asked Doreen to define autism, and Doreen said that it depended on the presence of three behavioural symptoms. These were social and language delay, and repetitive behaviour such as body rocking. We were on our way, with the interview consisting of the following questions and answers:

Sam to Doreen Granpeesheh: What is the link between autism and ADHD?

Children with ADHD, although not classified in the same chapter as the diagnostic criteria for autism, can have similar symptoms. Children with ADHD struggle to pay attention as do children with autism. It's difficult for children with ADHD to stay focused and therefore to learn.

Sam to Jeff Bradstreet: What are the causes of autism?

What we see is a normal period of development where no one feels concerned about the child's development and then all of a sudden, the child fades away, sometimes over a period of time and more often after three to four months, the family says he used to play with his siblings and doesn't do so anymore. He used to have language and eye contact and no longer has these skills. What causes this is a diverse group of environmental factors that may be impacting on genetic vulnerabilities. More often something in the environment triggers changes in the immune system, particularly in the brain functions. The immune system inside the brain is responsible for the building and design of the brain, as well as how the brain functions.

The getting of the symptoms part of autism is extremely complicated.

Some children may develop it from exposure to a toxin like lead or mercury. Another child may develop it from an immunological insult. Perhaps they got a really bad viral infection that triggered changes in their immune system. Those events can happen at any point in time, from inside Mom, to six months later, to 12 or 18 months later. When these events happen before three years of age and they generate the symptoms, then we'd call it autism.

Sam to Jeff Bradstreet: What does the Challenging Children Conference encompass?

We will be trying to integrate both the behavioural therapies and the diagnostic component of the biology and what you do once you diagnose the biology. We have found there are many things that can get the kids back on track. Sometimes it's treating gut or seizure disorder. Children can be remarkably restored to a much higher level of functioning.

Sam to Doreen Granpeesheh: Is autism on the increase?[7]

It is certainly on the increase. When I started in this field the incidence was 1 in 15 000 children in the United States. The current US statistics show that the incidence is now 1 in 150 children. It's an extremely high number.

Sam to Doreen Granpeesheh: What are the signs of autism?

A child around one year old should be able to start labelling single-word requests. Children with autism don't point to objects. This indicates that the child is missing an important skill called joint attention, which is the ability to hold your attention and indicate to you what they're think-ing. In their language development, the child with autism is not labelling objects or making requests. Some children aren't developing vocal language or [are developing] only limited vocal language. At two years old, a child should be describing things like 'big truck' or 'red car'. Children

---

7 Since this interview in 2009, the number has grown considerably. According to the Centers for Disease Control and Prevention in Atlanta, the figure for the United States it is now 1 in 59 children.

with autism may not go beyond the label 'car'. In some children, there is no speech; and in some there is speech but they're not using descriptive language.

Sam to Jeff Bradstreet: How did you get into your son Matthew's world?

Kids almost always have a specific interest. I always attach to what a particular child loves. Matthew had a fascination with dinosaur toys. We'd enter the child through the opening they gave us. This could be any obsessive interest that allows us in. If we look at the brain, those areas of the brain they're struggling with from a sensory processing point of view are areas we can now measure and see actual patho-physiology. There is inflammation and changes are taking place, which gives us access to quieten down what's happening in the brain abnormally. The therapists often tell us they see an acceleration in the child's ability to perform behaviourally or learn language. Working with ABA and biologically can be a very rewarding process.

Sam to Jeff Bradstreet: How do you calm down those inflamed areas biologically?

By using a variety of anti-inflammatories. These anti-inflammatories have been researched and studied and some have been reviewed and published. This is an exciting area of new development in treating autism.

My TV debut

The show then went to a commercial break. We were up next and went to sit on the couch with Sam. I think my face must have given away how scared I was. I could hear my heart pounding in my chest. The moment I sat down next to her, Sam tried to calm me down. She reassured me and told me to imagine that we were casually discussing David over a cup of coffee. She told me to look into her eyes and forget about the big black cameras across the room zooming in to focus.

We'd be going live in seconds and I heard the count down in the background – three, two, one … as we moved from the commercial break to being live on air. It was a surreal experience. Something I'd only read about or seen in a movie. Time stood still, but after answering the first question I became more confident.

Martin answered some questions also and Sam wanted to know what advice Martin had for other fathers going through a similar situation. Martin's advice won the hearts of everyone on set, including the viewers. He told Sam that he'd taken a decision to support his wife and be there for me no matter what, as I was the one who was in the face of the battle most of the time. During the next commercial break, Doreen told Martin that she had had cold shivers listening to him. When we got off the set and turned our phones back on, Martin's didn't stop beeping from friends and work colleagues congratulating him on being an outstanding father and exemplary husband.

I wasn't the same person walking off the set of *Great Expectations* as I had been walking on to it. Stepping out of my comfort zone and pushing myself beyond my perceived limits had paid off. It moulded the person I'd become and we'd been successful in reaching thousands of South African viewers with a very important message on autism. The message? That it was possible for children to move off the autism spectrum.

The Challenging Children Conference

I stood on stage beside Jeff Bradstreet. It was a proud moment as I gazed over the sea of people sitting in the auditorium. Dr Bradstreet asked me to open the conference and to introduce him to the audience. After all, it was fitting for the person who'd made all the arrangements to open the conference. I had no idea what I'd say as I held the microphone in my hand. Somehow, I found the words and welcomed everyone to the event I'd spent so much time conceptualising and organising. After the introduction, I went to take my seat in the front row close to the stage.

Jeff discussed the underlying medical causes for, and treatments of, autism. At tea break, a long queue formed around the hallway of the auditorium. Professionals stood around debating what they'd just learnt. I took a quick break outside and heard parents calling their families to tell them the good news that autism was a treatable medical illness. I saw tears streaming down their faces as they excitedly relayed the joyous message. The gasps and exclamations from the crowd said it all. I took a snapshot in my mind of the scene before me and savoured every moment. I was celebrating as I knew that the conference would have the desired outcome of changing the old school of thought I'd been exposed to for years – that autism was the end of the road. We'd already started to succeed in paving the way to healing for many autistic children.

It was lunchtime and I'd organised the doctors' lunch and Q & A with Jeff in a separate dining hall. He captivated his audience as the doctors in the room fired questions at him. A fierce debate ensued between him and one of the medical doctors who had for years been perceived as *the* authority on autism in South Africa. She'd sent children away from her consultations without even trying to treat the underlying causes; and was still prescribing only psychiatric medication to autistic children who were suffering from bowel disorders and a long list of treatable pathologies responsible for autism symptoms. She refused to accept what Jeff was telling her and strongly opposed the idea that autism was a treatable medical illness, sticking to her argument that these children were retarded. She snapped back at Jeff, insisting that the patients he was treating in his practice had to be different from the patients she was treating with psychiatric medication in her practice. I knew that her reluctance to accept the information presented had nothing to do with the truth, as Jeff had provided ample evidence and peer-reviewed papers in support of his claims. Whatever the reasons, she was desperately clinging to an old school of thought that was outdated and unfounded.

After lunch, Jeff resumed his presentation and showed further evidence supporting the fact that children with autism were immune-compromised and suffered from inflammation, impaired detoxification, nutrient deficiencies and that there was a gut–brain connection. He put forward one published paper after the next, with data to corroborate the findings on the causes and treatments.

What happened next was that several doctors, among them the woman who had previously been the 'only authority' on autism in South Africa, stormed out of the auditorium. They didn't like what they'd learnt, refusing to accept the evidence presented. It was clear to me that their decision to leave was motivated by their own personal agenda and that they hadn't considered the best interests of the children they claimed to represent.

Doreen Granpeesheh takes the stage next

It was time for Jeff to introduce Doreen, and he acknowledged her long list of credentials, achievements and awards for the enthusiastic crowd who'd been waiting in anticipation to hear her present on ABA.

Doreen has real stage presence. When she took the microphone, the audience hung on her every word. Doreen presented for hours on ABA, explaining the methodologies and strategies that were available to address different learning challenges and intermittently taking questions from an astonished audience. When she showed the documentary 'Recovered from Autism – A Journey through the Autism Spectrum and Back', you could hear a pin drop. Sadly for the four people who'd walked out after Jeff's presentation, they would miss what could have changed the way they viewed autism.

A way forward

The two-day conference ended on an exhilarating high, having provided renewed hope and inspiration to many. It had been everything I'd hoped it would be and more. We'd succeeded in changing the way autism would be perceived for decades to come in South Africa. I felt successful, and very hopeful about the future treatment of autism in our country.

Doreen had observed David at Little Stars the day before the conference, and had promised us a report and recommendations regarding his future education plan. She felt that David needed a communication device called a Dynavox; and that although he had potential, he needed an expert and an intensive ABA programme to get him back on track.

When I asked her which CARD office in America could accommodate us immediately, Doreen was silent for a few moments. 'Stay in your country,' she replied. 'I'll send one of my top clinical supervisors to South Africa to set up and manage an ABA programme for David. We'll come to you. Don't disrupt your life by moving to America.'

Doreen advised me to contact the psychology department at a local university. She suggested: 'Ask them if you can present to the final-year psychology students on ABA and autism. Once you've interviewed and selected a few students, CARD will help you train them in ABA. She added: 'I don't want people who *think* they know how to work with autistic children. I'm looking for young, energetic and intelligent psychology students who are passionate about working with children. It's for the same reasons students choose to study psychology that they will choose to be trained in ABA.' She explained further: 'ABA has its roots in the principles of psychology and students are always looking for practical experience, especially if they want to pursue a career in educational psychology.' I quickly saw the wisdom in what she was saying and was about to ask a couple of questions when Doreen caught me off guard by stating: 'In fact, I'm going to call Soo Cho right now and ask her to book herself a flight to South Africa.' There and then Doreen dialled Soo's number: 'Soo, I'm in South Africa. I have a parent sitting next to me. Her son is seven years old and you're going to fly to South Africa to set up and manage his ABA programme. Say hello to Ilana.'

Doreen handed me the phone and a surprised voice greeted me on the other end of the line. I could hear she was surprised, but I asked her when was the soonest she could come. She gave me a date two weeks from then, and undertook to book her ticket that very day. We ended the call with her asking me to complete the intake paperwork and send it to her in the meantime.

Jeff: our personal and national lifeboat

Jeff had confided in me that the autism epidemic could be likened to the devastating disaster of the *Titanic*. The world had not yet realised what a predicament and challenge autism would present to future generations. When the *Titanic* started to sink, very few people managed to get into the lifeboats to safety. However, after all we'd done for autism in South Africa, he'd ensure that we were secure on a national lifeboat and would also continue to help us restore David's health.

All I wanted was for my boy to speak. To hear his voice ... to know what he was feeling or thinking. Having endured deafening silence for too many years, I longed to communicate with him. Could there still be a chance that David would develop speech after all these years? That night when I said my prayers before bed, I fell on my knees on the floor and begged for mercy. Please, dear Lord, open the heavens to my prayers. From the depths of my soul, I desperately begged and prayed for David to be set free from the confines of the illness that debilitated him and impeded his ability to communicate. How long would he be chained to the shackles of the autism that imprisoned us both? After all, he was only a child and I a mother who'd endured the unthinkable. Most parents don't even think about the things I'd hoped and prayed for. When I eventually drifted off to sleep, I felt hopeful in the knowledge that Soo Cho would be arriving soon.

Saying goodbye to Doreen

The time had come to say goodbye to Doreen, and as we saw her off Martin asked her whether she'd have forgotten us by the time she arrived back home in America. He said that many people had promised their help over the years, but that very few had truly kept their promises. He wanted to know if she was going to be one of those people who made empty pledges. Unsurprisingly, Doreen was somewhat taken aback by Martin's comment but nevertheless undertook to keep her promise. As she walked away to board the plane, we held onto the hope of the assurance she'd given us.

Preparing for Soo's imminent arrival

As we prepared for Soo's arrival, every day brought new challenges. I'd presented the idea of converting Little Stars into a centre providing instructional ABA as a teaching methodology to our Little Stars teachers, and all ten of them opposed it. I had meetings with them to discuss their future and the transition to ABA, and all of them except one resigned, giving me short notice of their termination of employment. They'd all attended the conference and I was surprised by their resistance to change. However, I could not be deterred in my search to find a cure for David. After Doreen's trip, a light-bulb had been switched on in my brain. I clearly saw the route we needed to travel. Determined to get David onto a new path that would improve his quality of life and ours, I wasn't going to let a few resignations ruin my plans.

RECRUITING THE STUDENTS

I called the Department of Psychology at the University of Johannesburg, explained why I wanted to present to the students, and asked for an opportunity to address them. The head of department was very accommodating and set up a time for me to address the Honours class. I arrived outside the venue and waited anxiously for the class to fill up. I'd always feared presenting to crowds of people. I could easily conduct a round-table meeting, but standing in front of a room full of people made me feel intimidated and physically ill. I paused for a moment and took a deep breath. For a few seconds, as the students walked in to take their seats, the room started spinning around me. I felt dizzy and wanted to run away, but a voice inside forced me to stay and take control.

I asked the class whether they thought that autism was a lifelong disability. The students were in agreement that it was incurable. 'Are children with autism retarded?' I fired at the class. They all agreed that this was true. I took a question from one of the students, who wanted to know whether autistic children were bright, like Dustin Hoffman in the movie *Rain Man*. I continued to discuss the truths and myths about autism, clearing up the many misconceptions held about it. Then I appealed to the students for help and handed them a flyer so they could contact me for an interview. I wanted to gauge whether they were intrigued by my presentation; and so asked them to raise their hands if they were planning to contact me. A few arms went up reluctantly. I thanked the lecturer, turned around and made my way to the car in a hurry. It would soon be supper time and the kids were waiting for me. Driving home, I couldn't be sure that I'd been successful in achieving the goal Doreen had set me.

The next day, my phone didn't stop ringing. Most students in the class contacted me, wanting to find out the details. I booked time to interview them and hand-selected seven students for training. I had no recruitment team or set interview sheets to follow – all I had was Doreen's advice to find energetic young students who'd be passionate about working with autistic children. I learnt on the job and created my own interview procedures. I drafted employment contracts and wrote a code of conduct. I organised a first-aid course in anticipation of Soo's arrival and put in place all the pieces needed for the transition of Little Stars.

Soo touches down on South African soil

The only way I can properly describe Soo's arrival and first day of ABA training in South Africa is to conjure a desert scene. Before Soo and CARD we were lost in the desert, dragging our feet on the hot sand, bent over from exhaustion and heat. We had no compass, and no idea where we were going as the strong rays of the sun blinded our sight. One sandy hilltop blended into another. Near death, we lay helpless on the sand suffering from thirst and heat stroke. The vultures were circling, waiting for us to drop to the ground so they could pick away at our carcasses. When Soo arrived, it was like a big black chopper had appeared in the sky with an American flag emblazoned on the side. Down a rope came Soo, the American soldier with CARD's emblem on her uniform. Soo would rescue us from the desert storm, and provide the oasis we needed to end our pain and our wanderings.

That was precisely how I felt sitting through training on the first day of Soo's arrival in South Africa.

CHAPTER TEN

THE STAR ACADEMY

'Without language, one cannot talk to people and understand them; one cannot share their hopes and aspirations, grasp their history, appreciate their poetry, or savour their songs.' – Nelson Mandela

The jacaranda trees were in full bloom, colouring the Johannesburg skyline and creating a sea of purple petals on the streets. The blossoms created a magnificent, rich-purple carpet on our green lawn. Whenever I see the jacarandas in bloom, I'm reminded of Soo's arrival in our lives. More than anything else, because her trip brought colour into our son's gloomy grey world. She dipped her brush into a pot of ABA magic and painted David's world in colour.

Soo's interventions change all our lives

Soo had been sent to South Africa on a mission. Her brief was to turn David around. He was already seven years old, and we realised we were running out of time. But Doreen had kept her word and sent us Soo. We sat in our brand-new workshop area watching as Soo designed and worked out the details of David's education plan. David fought back, refusing to co-operate and demanding that everything be on his terms. Soo put his behaviour 'on extinction' and mapped out how we'd use the Dynavox – his new communication device, a gift from Doreen. This high-tech apparatus was quite heavy and had a sling attached to it so David could move around with it.

We marvelled over the Dynavox, having never seen anything like it before. That something like this actually existed was initially beyond our comprehension and imagination.

The idea behind the Dynavox was to teach David how to communicate effectively by using either the keyboard or the icons we'd specifically programmed for him. The device had different categories to choose from, including items David would need to ask for, such as food, clothes, people, locations and fun things to do. David would be able to push a button and communicate in a way that everyone would understand. Once he typed a word or chose a picture box, it would jump to the top of the screen. The device had voice output and would speak the word he'd chosen. Using the Dynavox would also result in his long-term independence. It was quite amazing!

We were never going to give up on teaching David vocal communication, but the Dynavox would be a way to give him a voice in the interim. It would alleviate his frustration by allowing him to communicate his needs and ask questions effectively.

LEARNING THAT LETTERS TOGETHER MAKE WORDS

David had always been fascinated by letters, words and the alphabet. He'd walk up to a wall-poster with words on it or find words in a book, and he'd run his hand over them, closely studying the letters. It was the same when we went shopping in Woolworths, where the trolley we were pushing around featured the store's name in large letters. David ran his hand slowly over each one, and I knew he was curious about what the word meant. What I didn't know then was how to use his interest in the alphabet effectively to help him communicate.

Soo had the training and experience to turn David's love for written words and letters into functional communication. We now came to realise that David understood more than we'd thought he did. For all these years, he'd wanted to share so many things but had had no way of telling us. With the new device, it became possible for David to have a voice. In no time, he learnt to communicate. He quickly acquired hundreds of words he could use to 'speak' to us (and which he could even spell). For the first time in seven years David was able to tell us what he wanted, where he wanted to go, what his favourite colour was and when he wanted to engage in certain activities. The Dynavox changed his life and ours. It was heart-warming to watch him break into a smile when he had successfully put his thoughts across or managed to ask for a specific person or item. David fell asleep and woke up with the Dynavox in his hand. It became his voice and he carried it around day and night.

Because we'd given him an effective means of communication, David's challenging behaviours began to manifest less often, and his ABA graphs for aggression, tantrums and self-injurious behaviour began to come down. If we could get him to learn that he could use his device all the time to communicate instead of trying to gain our attention through bad behaviour, we could get rid of the crying and screaming that so often resonated throughout the house. It's one thing for a two- or three-year-old to cry and scream in order to get their point across, but a seven-year-old engaging in this behaviour is another story. I also knew it wouldn't go away unless David learnt another way to communicate.

A WALL OF WORDS

We began to base our approach on David spontaneously using the Dynavox as his first go-to when he wanted to say something, and in no time he became quite proficient at employing the device.

There was only one drawback to the Dynavox. It was very heavy, and this made it really tough for David to carry to the shops or the park. We safeguarded the machine as if it were another child. It had to be charged morning and evening, and one of the members of David's team became responsible for programming it and adding to it every new word David learnt. This was nail-biting stuff as he couldn't be without it – not even for a minute. We had to back it up and sometimes it froze and would need to be restarted. We also had to watch that David didn't drop it.

Eli was so proud of David's new abilities that he begged me on numerous occasions to be allowed to take his older brother to school to show off to his friends. It was a phenomenon to watch David using the communication programme: for a child who'd struggled so much to produce vocal words, we were astounded at what he could tell us through his Dynavox. Obviously, his extensive vocabulary had been buried deep inside him for years and was now bursting to come out.

It's important to note here that a child's autism has nothing to do with their IQ; and that, in fact, an autistic child often has an extremely high IQ. Just because they can't give you the vocal output doesn't mean all the information isn't stored on their internal hard drive. The problem for an autistic child is finding a way of putting out the fire in their brain, then renovating the wiring needed to retrieve the stored information.

DAVID'S DYNAVOX VOICE

David could navigate through the different pages and screens like a trained pilot who knew what to do with every button on his control panel. It was incredible to watch how fast he'd go in and out of the different options looking for the icon or word he wanted to use. Doreen *had* succeeded in giving David a voice.

When David asked for something on his Dynavox, we made sure to comply with his requests immediately so he could learn that the device was a way to get what he wanted. In time we'd fade this rush to get him what he wanted or to jump in the car and take him to a location immediately. In the real world that's not always possible and over time David had to learn he couldn't always get what he asked for straight away. We had to introduce David to the concept that he couldn't always just ask and be obeyed. For example, wanting to go to the park at 9 pm just wasn't an option and he had to fall in with the rest of the family's schedule and with obvious safety considerations. That was yet another step on the road to David becoming both independent and integrated ...

THE MISSING DYNAVOX OR THE WORST HOUR OF MY LIFE

I'll never forget the day I lost the magical Dynavox. I had decided to take David shopping with me. When we arrived at the mall, I placed him and his Dynavox inside the trolley as I'd done on numerous occasions. I became lost in my own world of shopping and soon the trolley was filled to the top with parcels from various stores. I was already on my way to the car when

I realised the Dynavox was missing. Panic overcame me as I raced over to the information desk. By this time I was already crying, battling to get the words out as I explained to the lady sitting behind the desk that my son was autistic and that I'd lost his Dynavox – his voice! She must have thought I was crazy as I frantically begged for her help in trying to locate the device.

She called security and the hunt for the Dynavox began. I raced from shop to shop, flustered and desperate to find the Dynavox. As I have explained, it was very expensive and essential to David's functioning and happiness. On top of that, it wasn't insured at the time! As I made my way to the toy store where we'd shopped earlier, a security guard came running after me, waving the device. David had placed it on one of the shelves at the toy store without my noticing. Beyond grateful, I thanked the guard and made my way back to the car. It had all been just too much and I sobbed the whole way home.

In later years, the iPad revolutionised what is called 'augmentative communication'. We were able to replace the Dynavox with an iPad and a communication app called TouchChat which replicated the Dynavox and made it obsolete. I'd like to caution parents and professionals not to judge a child's ability by their lack of vocal communication. Once a child is taught how to use an appropriate means of communication such as TouchChat, a whole new world opens for everyone involved.

COUNTING DOWN THE MEANING OF TIME

Soo's behaviour-intervention plan also made it possible for us to stand in line at the shops. Something as simple as queuing, which most people take for granted, had become impossible for me and David as he'd become frustrated and irritable if the line didn't move fast enough.

Soo explained that David didn't understand the concept of time and put in place a timer I could take with me everywhere to *show* David what time meant. This new method drastically changed my trips to the mall. As we entered the line at Woolworths, I'd tell David we'd be there for 15 minutes and then turn on the timer so he could watch the seconds tick by. When the alarm went off, he'd know that 15 minutes had come to an end and that it was time to go.

There was only one drawback to using a timer: if the device went off, I'd have to leave immediately to honour what I had told David before setting the clock. So I'd always add an extra five minutes in case the person in front of me took longer than expected. We also used this method if we were out at a restaurant or any other public place. David would become anxious about how long we were going to be somewhere, and didn't understand if we simply told him 'five more minutes'. Yet when we gave him a timer that counted down the five minutes, he'd understand the abstract concept of time. The timer prevented David from having a meltdown in public, making going out much easier for us as a family.

Soo's widespread impact on autism in South Africa

With David settled on the Dynavox, we took a closer look at his vocals. Soo decided that it would be a good time to get the PROMPT programme going again for David. We agreed that PROMPT incorporated into an ABA programme would be the best combination for David. This time around I'd have a team to support me; and if we delivered PROMPT to David at regular intervals daily, we stood a chance of being successful. In future years at The Star Academy, this combination would open up a world of speech for many children who passed through our doors.

Soo designed programmes for four other children besides David. The week went by in a flash. Soo had trained the psychology students I had recruited in the knowledge and skills of ABA, and now assigned them in teams to David and four other children. The plan was for Soo to manage and supervise the programme remotely from the United States, and we set a date for her return to South Africa three months later.

For the next three years, Soo came back to South Africa for one week every three months. On each visit she placed another five children on our The Star Academy programme, which was the foundation from which the Academy grew. The Star Academy had officially become an affiliate of CARD – one of only a few in the world and the only one in Africa.

Since its inception, the Academy has continued to excel in providing ABA programmes to children on the continent. Working with our core team, Soo imparted her knowledge to such an extent that the team was able to set up satellite academies in South Africa and elsewhere, reaching children in Ghana, Zimbabwe, Mauritius and Rwanda.

Another result of Soo's initial visit was the implementation of daily Skype observations by her CARD support team. Despite the different time zones, CARD's dedicated staff watched over both our junior and our senior instructors, guiding them every step of the way. This sometimes meant they worked until past midnight – a good lesson for our staff on what dedication really means.

Six months on from Soo's first visit, there was such a demand for ABA that Doreen decided to add another clinical supervisor, Brian White, to help with the caseload. His appointment and years of experience added a whole new dimension to our staff training.

Soaking up Soo's and Brian's expertise

Soo and Brian can only be described as Doreen's 'big guns'. When either one visited us, Martin and I would find ourselves working and learning from them – often until 2 or 3 am. We knew it was as important for them as it was for us to know that we were running The Star Academy to their incredibly high standards.

Such was our success that we found ourselves having to recruit new instructors every two or three months to meet the growing demand for ABA. Naturally, these instructors needed to walk the same intense route as that followed by our initial team. Whenever Brian or Soo were here, they covered the spectrum of issues our instructors faced on a daily basis as part of their staff training.

By 2010 we'd grown from 5 to 25 children, each with a different set of deficits requiring tailor-made education plans to address their needs. It's important to remember that when we talk of a 'child with autism', the term is so broad as to not really be useful. The autism spectrum in fact encompasses a very wide variety of children, ranging from those who have no vocal expression to those who possess a particularly advanced command of language but nevertheless struggle with a deficit somewhere in their skill set. However competent they may appear on the surface, even these children would battle in a mainstream school setting without an ABA programme to support them.

CHAPTER ELEVEN

YEAR TWO: MAKING OUR MARK

As David was now rapidly gaining skills for everyday life, Martin and I could take a breather for the first time in years. We were now feeling more hopeful about what our future might hold. Despite this shift, however, I threw myself into The Star Academy, running away from all my buried sadness and regularly working way past midnight.

Doreen kept her promise to return to South Africa and we were extremely proud to show her what we'd established with her help. I spent another year organising a second Challenging Children Conference. This time Doreen would partner with Dr Brian Jepson. He would lecture on possible medical interventions in autism and Doreen – of course – would present on the educational and behavioural aspects of treatment.

Again the event was very successful, bringing answers to so many desperate people – parents, families and professionals alike. They flocked to the sessions, coming away with the answers they so eagerly sought. We continued to send shock waves throughout the South African autism community, dispelling the archaic beliefs that had been in place for so long. With this conference too, the demand for ABA grew. We had to try to cope with the need and would have meeting after meeting putting systems, programmes and more infrastructure in place for desperate parents.

The Star Academy spreads its wings

PRETORIA, 2011

Because parents were driving for over an hour each way from Pretoria to Johannesburg and back to bring their children to what had now become an expert unit, we took the decision to set up a similar academy in Pretoria.

Soon thereafter, I found myself at the University of Pretoria to recruit psychology students. This time I didn't bother to go the 'official' route – I just barged into their lecture, with David and his Dynavox in tow. I asked graciously whether the psychology professor would give me five minutes to talk to the class. He took one look at David and found himself unable to refuse his crazy mother.

I was pressed for time and under pressure; and had to choose my words very carefully in order to grab the students' attention. I summarised the key issues that define autism. I also explained the life of a parent living with autism and the need for ABA instruction. When I asked for a show of hands to see who was going to apply, I had a good response. When I interviewed the students, they all told me that seeing David with his angelic face communicate through his Dynavox had encouraged them to apply. After one week of interviews, I had my Pretoria team.

Within a few weeks we'd secured a location and were up and running with our first five children. Over the years the Pretoria Academy has grown and has become an essential lifeline for parents in and around the area.

Durban, 2012

The Durban Academy had its beginnings in 2010, when a medical doctor living in that city found me on the internet after his two-year-old son was diagnosed with autism. I flew to Durban and addressed the psychology students at the University of KwaZulu-Natal. By now I was getting the hang of talking to psychology students! A few weeks later, we opened a bright and sunny new academy in Umhlanga that became a beacon of hope for many parents.

Reaching families across South Africa

As each enquiry came in from families throughout South Africa, we'd find a way to help them.

Today we work with families in Rustenburg, Hartbeespoort Dam, Potchefstroom, Tzaneen, Port Shepstone and Makhanda (Grahamstown). We regularly send our instructors and supervisors to their homes to help them train their own local instructors and from time to time they visit our academies in Johannesburg and Pretoria.

Training the staff as Board Certified Autism Technicians

It was during one of our calls with Doreen that she happened to mention her New York office would be sitting for a new certification in ABA. She suggested it would be a good idea to have our South African instructors take the exam.

Within an hour of our call I'd received all the information we needed to take the first-ever Board Certified Autism Technician (BCAT) exam. The BCAT credential was created by the Behavioral Intervention Certification Council (BICC) – the first and so far only autism-specific credential accredited by the National Commission for Certifying Agencies (NCCA).

The mission of the BICC is to 'enhance public protection by developing and administering a certification programme consistent with the needs of behaviour analysis to recognise individuals who are qualified to treat the deficits and behaviours associated with autism spectrum disorder using the principles and procedures of applied behaviour analysis.'

With 100 Academy staff members and only five days to prepare, we came face to face with the 40 hours of video training the exam required us to cover. Our team had to continue with their normal work during the day as we couldn't cancel our scheduled sessions with the children, and would thus have to study late into the night to get through the coursework. At the time, South Africa was having regular power cuts. In addition, not everyone had the luxury of a fast internet line at home. To say we panicked is putting it mildly.

MAKING IT HAPPEN DESPITE THE ODDS

I knew I had to find a way to prepare our team properly. We divided the coursework into sections so we'd have summaries of the material we had to cover. One of the CARD trainers made herself available to us on Skype and in three hours covered as much material as she could to prepare everyone.

Preparing for the exam wasn't the only stumbling block. We had to organise an exam venue and proctors who would make themselves available to supervise the exam. These had to be people we didn't know. They had to sign forms in which they committed to be impartial and responsible for the exam supervision. This wasn't easy to arrange, especially on short notice. After a number of calls, I thought of asking the University of Pretoria for help. They obliged and we made contact with the selected proctors to get them to sign all the necessary forms. Arrangements for Johannesburg and Pretoria were covered, but we still needed to finalise arrangements for Durban and our other African affiliates' instructors. Nevertheless, all our instructors presented themselves to sit for the three-hour BCAT exam – all of them part of making history.

The exam papers were collected and shipped to the United States, and we waited in anticipation for the marks to be released. Late one Saturday evening, two weeks after the exam, the email with the news arrived in my inbox. I was afraid to read it and hoped I'd be sharing good news with everyone. We achieved a 98 per cent overall pass rate with many high distinctions. The congratulations poured in as The Star Academy team excitedly shared the good news on social media and went out to celebrate. Not only had we achieved the golden standard of approval: we had also passed with flying colours.

By requiring all its staff to obtain and maintain the BCAT credential, The Star Academy assures that its children are receiving an international standard of treatment from responsible, accountable and regulated professionals.

FOLLOWING MY STAFF MEMBERS' EXAMPLE

I now had a burning desire to take the BCAT exam myself. If I were to earn the respect of my team, I had to prove to them that I too could become certified. The only time I had available to cover the coursework was at 4 am in the morning, before I got the kids out the door and ready for school; or from 11 pm at night, after replying to my emails and cleaning the kitchen. I sat up late, night after night. A number of years had passed since I'd written an exam and I was quite nervous as I waited to begin the paper online. I did it, and passed with flying colours.

The jewel in our crown: The Yellow Canaries Project, Tembisa, 2015

'Each of us as citizens has a role to play in creating a better world for our children.' – Nelson Mandela

Tembisa is a large township that is home to many underprivileged South Africans. Situated to the north of Kempton Park in Ekurhuleni, Gauteng, it was established in 1957 when black people were resettled there from other underprivileged areas. '*Thembisa*' is an Nguni word meaning 'promise' or 'hope'. In the case of The Star Academy's involvement in this community, the name turned out to be appropriate.

In 2015 the Academy received a call from Tembisa Hospital's psychology team, whose members wanted to learn more about ABA and the possibility of supporting the parents of autistic children living in the surrounding community. The team was being approached by more and more parents seeking its help. In search of solutions, it wanted to meet with me to discuss the options available and how it could enhance the therapies it already provided.

At our first meeting at our offices with the psychologist who represented the team, I was moved as I listened to stories concerning parents in the area raising children with autism. I was told about mothers having to walk for over an hour to the hospital to seek help for their autistic children. The patients were receiving speech and occupational therapy for a mere 45 minutes once a week, and the psychologists were finding it quite a challenge to work through many of the behavioural issues they were coming across.

Struggling to survive, each day these mothers face many stumbling blocks, including that of feeding their children adequately. Autistic children can be picky eaters, which makes good nutrition really hard when you're on a tight budget. Not only do their mothers not always have money for the very basics – such as a roof over their heads and food on their tables – but they are also dealing with the long list of struggles autism presents.

This first meeting with the Tembisa psychologist, therefore, was a very sobering experience for me. I had believed for so long that I had an extremely difficult life and that I'd been dealt a terrible blow in having to tussle with autism. The meeting changed my perspective on how bad my life truly was, and I promised to schedule a time to meet with her head of department and the rest of her team at the hospital.

Very soon after this initial meeting, I made my way to the township. Driving there, I wondered how we could help the parents of Tembisa and alleviate their burden. As I arrived, Annah Motshatama, a recently employed instructor at The Star Academy who lived in Tembisa, greeted me at the entrance to the hospital. I'd asked her to come with me to the meeting as I thought it a good idea to get her involved in this project, considering she lived in the area.

I felt nervous and totally unprepared walking with Annah to meet the psychology team. I'd forgotten my pen and paper in the car and I'd rushed out the door that morning looking barely decent. Putting on make-up is never on my agenda as there's simply no time for frills. I straightened my clothes and smoothed my hair with my hands, remembering that I'd run out of time to brush it. 'How do I look?' I asked Annah, who was dressed to perfection and immaculate. As she grinned, I thought: 'To hell with it, I'm going to blow them away with my ideas and passion to find them solutions – even though I look as if I just climbed out of the washing basket!'

As we reached the boardroom and the whole team greeted me, I prayed silently that I would come up with a way to help everyone. All eyes and ears were on me, waiting to see and hear what I had to say about autism treatment and a solution.

I had given some thought to the treacherous daily battle Tembisa parents were fighting, and spoke to the team about the potential benefits of ABA. They were open to the idea, and I explained that I'd have my staff train their team in behaviour management and other skills, making it easier for them to deliver their therapy.

137

BRINGING SOME 'STAR' MAGIC TO TEMBISA

On the way home, I called Martin from the car. 'We have to help these families!' I implored him. Blessed with all the support and access to anything and everything we had ever needed, I wanted to help parents who weren't so lucky. I could only try to imagine the horror they endured daily. Martin gave me his assurance that we wouldn't walk away from their plight; and agreed that we had a responsibility to improve their lives. We both understood that helping other families was the glue necessary to mend our broken hearts.

I got back to my office and called *The Tembisan* to place an advert looking for students to train in ABA. In no time, the phone rang off the hook as I fielded calls from willing students and young Tembisa residents who wanted to be trained in ABA. I must have interviewed 50 students before I selected the top ten applicants. I set a date for their ABA training at The Star Academy and put in place everything we needed to bring them up to speed.

On the first day of training I welcomed the group and gave them an inspiring talk on autism and why ABA was such a powerful tool. I explained how it would change the lives of the children they'd be working with. I remember looking around the room at the eager young faces who were so happy to be chosen to work on this project. By training these students, not only were we going to help the autistic children of Tembisa: we would also be creating jobs. Training kicked off. Next on my list was finding funding for the project!

THE YELLOW CANARIES OF TEMBISA IS ESTABLISHED

We decided to name the Tembisa outreach programme the Yellow Canaries Project. We hoped that the colourful name would draw the attention and interest of the public in the area. We also knew, from past experience, that people always find the facts behind the name arresting – something to ponder about.

The hospital provided us with a stand-alone, prefabricated container to work from. With trained staff and enough funding to get the programme off the ground, we enrolled the first ten children. One of The Star Academy

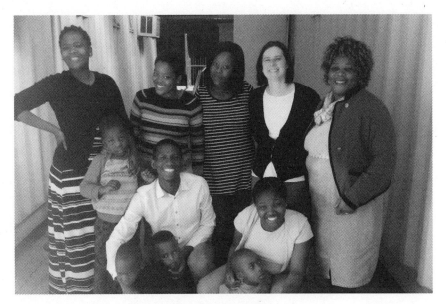

The Tembisa team

case managers designed and managed the programmes. The newly trained students delivered the individualised education plans under the supervision of a long-time staff member with over 20 years' experience in working with children with autism. This was Lizzie Mabasa, who had worked for me when we opened Little Stars, and now agreed to relocate to Tembisa to manage the new team.

MUCH-NEEDED SUPPORT FOR PARENTS
Together with the psychology department of Tembisa Hospital, we established a parent-support group. This was intended to give parents an opportunity to share their hardships; and to ask questions about managing the complex diagnosis of autism and its many demands.

A frequent issue raised in these meetings was how family and extended family members would mock the autistic child, not understanding why the child couldn't speak or communicate like other children.

CHICKEN SOUP REALLY IS MEDICINE!
Whether you live in Tembisa or the affluent area of Sandton, the worries

139

and struggles of parents of autistic children are the same. Fear of the future and a longing to hear their children's voices was evident from my encounters with Tembisa parents. Toilet training was top of their agenda. They also wanted to know what to feed their children and if diet played a role. Talking to families whose food budget was limited, I had to be very creative in my advice. It wasn't as if they could just pop over to an upmarket shop to purchase some gluten-free products. In a community where the staple foods were maize and milk, it was going to be difficult to suggest a rotational and dairy-free diet. (Children on the autism spectrum can suffer from food allergies. For this reason, alternating proteins daily is recommended to avoid these allergies.)

In the end, the answer to the problem was easy – as long as they had freezers at home. They could all make chicken and beef soup; and then freeze them in smaller or larger batches.

WHATSAPP CONVERSATION BETWEEN BEATRICE, ONE OF THE TEMBISA MUMS, AND ILANA

B: Good day, this is how my beef and chicken broth came out. On top are some fats and the second layer is like spicy stock and under it's a broth gel. My question is should I take out the fats and spice and only use the broth gel. Thanks.

I: Don't take anything out. Give it all. So proud of u. It looks delicious and amazing!!!!!! And I love how u have it in glass jars. That's wonderful. Better to store in glass rather than plastic if possible as plastic can breed bacteria.

B: Thank you, I will start feeding him tonight. I want to thank you guys, from 3 months ago, or let me say from since my son was a little boy, for the first time today we had hard yellow non-smelling poo. I thank you very much for the advice and support. I think beef and chicken broth and chicken soup is our new family lifestyle.

I: Yay – U r an inspiration. So proud of u. More to come. Always hope. Keep fighting.

B: Thank you I was out of options. We will continue to fight till we've solved the puzzle.

ANGRY ANCESTORS

Our very first Tembisa student was a three-year-old boy whose mother had abandoned him after realising something was wrong and he wasn't reaching his milestones on time. She noticed he wasn't able to speak and left him with his father at their home in Tembisa, never to return. She was afraid, scared and felt helpless. His father, having to work and put food on the table, took him to his grandmother in a rural area to raise him while he worked to pay the bills. The other children in this community began to laugh at him and mocked him for being unable to speak. In desperation, his grandmother took him to the local traditional healer to ask for a remedy. The traditional healer noted that the ancestors were in all likelihood angry with this child and decided to cut his wrists until he bled in the hope of making him talk. When the bleeding didn't produce results, his father took him to Tembisa Hospital, where he was introduced to the Yellow Canaries Project.

This is just one of many stories of parents who were subjected to communities who misunderstood autism and had no idea how to treat it.

BRINGING HOPE TO FAMILIES IN TEMBISA
– NICOLE MOODLEY, BCAT

'The progress at Tembisa has been an incredible journey. The Yellow Canaries outreach programme does more than just bring quality ABA to families – it brings about a new sense of hope and faith [to parents] that their child now has a fighting chance. These families have seen tremendous progress since we started the Tembisa programme two years ago. It's wonderful to witness parents so dedicated to their children, regardless of the limitations that come with autism. These parents go above and beyond for their children. We've had parents with very little achieve great things.

'One of the biggest challenges facing these families is the affordability of specialised diets. But we have moms who use their limited resources to provide healthier alternatives – for example bone broth – for their kids. This to me lets other parents know there's always a way – irrespective of all the limitations.

'I've begun facilitating the parents' support group and parent training. The meetings address issues and concerns from parents in the programme and those on the waiting list. It's great to see how many parents have grown within the group and in turn impact others around them.

'The parents' support group helps them navigate their lives within a learning environment that equips their children to [reach] their best potential. The parents that attend the support group inspire other parents, encouraging each other to be the best caregiver they can for their kids.

'With these support groups, I've had the opportunity to glance into and understand what happens after these kids leave their ABA setting. The trials and tribulations of these parents have inspired me to become a better instructor and I've gained a great wealth of knowledge from the perspective of the parent/caregiver.

'This is just the beginning of creating more awareness and education around autism. The wheels have begun to change in communities previously uninformed about autism, and it's a great opportunity for The Star Academy to be at the forefront of this endeavour.

'The dedication of the parents of the Yellow Canaries has proven that with awareness and a 'no excuses' mindset they can bring about meaningful change in their child's life. I've truly seen the inner strength of parents despite the odds against them.'

ANNAH MOTSHATAMA, BCAT
'I love kids but what particularly appealed to me about working at The Star Academy was the opportunity to spread the word on autism treatment, as there's so much information out there that people don't know about. I'm from a township where I've seen a lot of kids with these symptoms – so I wanted to help bring awareness and access to people.'

The Yellow Canaries Project
'In 2015 I helped to start The Star Academy's project in Tembisa. There's a long list of children who need help in the area and at present, due to lack of funding, our reach is limited.

'What has made a big difference though is the parents' support group. Here they can get help and information from a multi-disciplinary group.'

Overcoming cultural issues
'Unfortunately, in these areas, there are also a lot of stereotypes [and people] who think that if their child has a medical or behavioural problem they've been bewitched or something similar. Through us arming them with knowledge, more and more parents are getting to understand autism. With support groups and sharing, I do believe we're starting to make a difference.'

A light at the end of the tunnel
'The parents feel trapped but they trust us and we give them help and hope. We teach them how to interact and play with their children at home so they can relate better and have normal, natural interaction. For me it's been a life-changing experience. They now tell us their child comes to them when they call them; their child can now be potty-trained. It's the small things most people take for granted. It's life-changing when you're part of this and I love it.

'My dream would be to expand The Yellow Canaries Project. It's heartbreaking to turn people away, although our parents' support group does fill that void.'

CHAPTER TWELVE

A LEAP OF FAITH

In the two years from when we'd established The Star Academy in 2009, David had made measurable progress. He could now communicate effectively using his Dynavox, and although his vocals were slow there was progress. During these two years David's behaviour settled, he became able to sustain his attention for longer periods of time and learning was taking place. His health was improving, especially his gut health, and life had become a little more settled.

It had been a long and hard eight years since David's autism diagnosis. There was never a day, hour, minute or second when I didn't carry around a deep feeling of pain and loss. Navigating my life through the agony of pain and suffering was something that was ongoing. We were still moving mountains to transform David's autism into a state of remission. I felt incomplete and empty, even after clawing my way out of the deepest and most unimaginable darkness. We longed for another child and consulted our experts in the United States. Hours of research later, we concluded that there was a 50 per cent risk of having another child with autism. But although we weighed the risk, our longing for another child overshadowed all our doubts. We were confident that this time around we knew enough to avoid losing a child to this insidious illness. We had a burning desire to bring more joy into our life to overshadow the grief, and we simply had more to give. Very soon after taking the decision to go ahead with our plan of extending our family, we were expecting another child.

Joy mixed with fear

We didn't share the news of my pregnancy with anyone until I was six months along. When we eventually told friends and family they were relieved, having wondered why I'd put on weight but not wanting to pry or say the wrong thing. I simply couldn't talk about it, afraid to jinx the outcome. I had deep feelings of concern over the decision but tried to bury the worry somewhere safe in my subconscious, carrying on with my daily tasks and keeping myself occupied at work.

At around six months into the pregnancy I went for a scan to check on the baby's sex. The doctor confirmed it was a boy. I swallowed hard, knowing that this would only increase the long list of dangers we faced relating to my pregnancy and the baby's future. Once again, I buried the voice inside me that kept reminding me of the risks we were taking.

Aaron is born, 30 May 2012

Nine months of a normal pregnancy flew past. I checked into the maternity ward afraid but hoping for the best as I once again prepared myself for a scheduled Caesarean section. We were extremely nervous and worried about any complications that might arise. If there were any, we'd have to take quick and smart decisions at that moment. We had a medical expert from America on call waiting on the other end of the telephone to guide us in case we needed him. Lying on the metal table waiting for the doctor to arrive to deliver Aaron was nail-biting stuff. I watched the clock on the wall and felt the surgeon tug on my lower belly as he made the incision. In no time, I heard a baby crying and the paediatrician whisked the baby away to do the normal Apgar tests in the corner of the room. I turned my head to watch and when I saw Aaron for the first time my heart dropped. I felt cold and I couldn't believe what I'd seen.

I was looking at the spitting image of David. Uneasiness overwhelmed me and I felt an ominous feeling in my heart. Even though I'd had a spinal block and the doctor was sewing me up, I was fully aware of everything around me. I had great clarity of mind … and was fighting for control of my faculties as hard as I could.

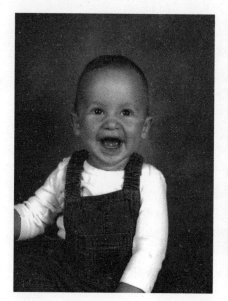 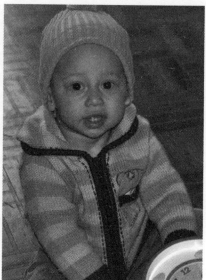

David and Aaron as newborns

This can't be happening again …

The paediatrician walked over and handed the baby to me. I held Aaron for the first time and when I looked at his little wrinkled face staring back at me all I could think of was how much he looked like David. I fought back the tears and thanked the paediatrician. The Apgar score was nine out of ten and the paediatrician assured me his breathing and skin tone were perfect. He was happy with his overall appearance and as far as he was concerned there was no reason to worry. The nurse placed Aaron back in the incubator and wheeled me into the recovery room. I had to make sure Aaron would latch and breastfeed. Even though I felt a little woozy, I kept reminding myself to concentrate and tried to overcome the drowsiness I was feeling. I raised his head and guided him to latch onto my breast but he wasn't latching. 'Why is he not latching?' I screamed, and summoned the nurse to help me. She reassured me that he'd latch and tried to calm me down. Aaron didn't latch on his first day of life and neither had David.

This time around, I knew that colostrum (secreted by a mother's breasts close to the time of birth) was important for gut health, contributing as it does to the development of the microbiome that is key to ensuring a healthy gut flora. I squeezed out the colostrum onto a spoon and watched as the nurse helped me to get Aaron to swallow it. I breathed a sigh of relief and fell asleep. The next day, and after much encouragement, Aaron latched on.

Martin brought David and Eli to the hospital to meet the new addition to the Gerschlowitz family. Eli was excited to hold his new brother and David was drawn to the little baby lying in the bassinet crying his lungs out. All our attention was directed at Aaron and it felt as if we were taking a break from autism for just a short moment in time. I refused vaccines, to the utter dismay of my paediatrician, who vowed not to sign my release forms if I didn't consent to them. He eventually had no choice but to honour my decision.

From the moment I brought Aaron home, I watched over him night and day. I guarded him 24 hours a day, like a soldier standing guard and scanning the environment for danger. I slept beside him and was extremely careful what baby creams, shampoos or medication I used for him.

The days rolled into weeks, and as the months passed, Aaron developed perfectly, reaching all his milestones. This wasn't enough to reassure me, however, as David had done the same.

I remember when Aaron copied me waving goodbye. Imitation as a skill was present early on and I was bursting with pride at his first babbling sounds of mama and dada. I have pictures of him pointing to his birthday cake when he turned one.

Celebration and sadness

It was 30 May 2013 and Aaron's first birthday. Sadly, this happy occasion coincided with my father's sudden death from a heart attack. We'd just gone to bed having celebrated Aaron's birthday when, just after midnight, my mother called with the bad news that my dad had passed away.

The next morning, Aaron woke up crying and irritable from an ear infection. It would be the first of many ear infections to follow. Trying to avoid oral antibiotics, I used a topical ear drop instead, coupled with homeopathic remedies. Later in the day, we took the long drive home to

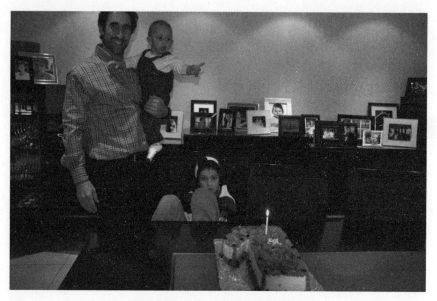

Aaron pointing at his first birthday cake

Kestell for my father's burial. Since we'd be away the whole day, we decided to take David with us. In the car on the way there, I was unsure about our decision as David would have to accompany us to the gravesite. He was only ten years. By the time we arrived in Kestell, however, I had pushed aside the ominous and uneasy feelings that had made me so unsettled, and David attended the funeral.

In the car on the way, I decided that I needed to see my father before he was buried. I needed closure. I arrived at the cemetery and, as I came closer to the tiny brick structure that served as the room where the body was prepared for burial, two men approached me. I told them that I *had to* see my father but was told in a matter-of-fact tone that this would not be possible as they had already nailed the coffin shut. 'Well then,' I told them, 'you'll be opening the coffin and undoing the nails'.

I walked up the broken staircase to the room where the coffin had been placed on a small metal table. The room was dark with cobwebs and the light stealing in through the broken windowpane was sparse. A candle burned next to the coffin. In Jewish tradition, the candle represents the dead person's soul and must be kept alight until the body is buried.

I stood next to the coffin as the two men used a hammer to pry it open. Within a few minutes they had lifted the lid, and I saw my father for the first time since hearing the news of his passing. Standing in that room was a life-changing experience for me. In that moment, as I looked at my father's lifeless body, I knew for certain that there existed a physical body and a separate soul. It was now all very clear to me: the natural thing to do was to put the body in the ground; my father had left and was no longer in our physical world.

Viewing his body brought me immense closure and peace of heart. The two men left to give us time alone. I studied my father's lifeless hands and remembered how I'd clutch onto them as a little girl when he took me to the park. Standing next to him, I connected with him on a spiritual level and whispered to him softly. I knew he had been waiting for me to come. 'Daddy, I'm here – I'm so sorry … Please go up to heaven,' I encouraged him. 'Don't be afraid, Daddy – I'm here now – you can go.'

The men returned, closed the lid and sealed the coffin anew. As I walked away from them and from my father's body towards the people assembled for the funeral, I had no tears left to shed.

Family and friends were called to accompany the body to the grave. One by one they came forward as their names were called, to pay my father their last respects and carry the coffin to the open grave. I looked in my brother's direction as the coffin was carefully lowered into the ground. He was bent over and was crying. As the first thud of fresh soil landed on the coffin lid, his loud cries echoed through the silent cemetery. My heart went out to him and I realised that viewing the body before burial was the best thing I could have done: I knew that my father's soul had departed; and was thus able to accept that his body belonged to the ground.

Everyone took turns to cover the coffin with soil and, as we turned to leave, the congregation made two rows on either side of the grave to allow the mourners to walk away first. I was looking down at the dusty path as I made my way back to the brick structure where I'd viewed the coffin, when I heard the footsteps of a man who was running behind me. He started calling my name insistently, over and over. I stopped and turned around as he caught up to me. With a firm handshake, he introduced himself as my father's attorney and the executor of his last Will and testament. I noticed he was clutching a white envelope to his chest.

Still out of breath, he told me it was urgent that we speak and asked if I'd be willing to accompany him to his office. I wondered what could be so urgent at a time like this – the soil covering my father's coffin was still fresh. Although reluctant at first to disclose the full reason for his request, he volunteered that my father had signed a new Will a few weeks before and that there were things I needed to know as an adjunct to this.

I gathered up Martin and David, briefly explained the situation, and we followed the attorney to his office. The streets were deserted and the journey was a rapid one. We entered his office and sat down on big brown couches. Martin, David and I sat facing him, curiously awaiting what he had to say. He began by describing how my father had confided in him that he'd struggled to help us with David's autism. My father had felt that he'd failed us by not knowing how to help us during his lifetime. He wanted to make sure that, in his death, he would be able to make amends by creating a special trust fund for David.

Ten minutes later, we found ourselves in the car driving back to Johannesburg. Martin and I had tears streaming down our faces. My father's gesture had touched us very deeply. Our relationship with him had been strained for many years. He'd simply not known how to give us the emotional support we'd so desperately needed, especially in the early years of our battle with autism. In his death, he'd succeeded in showing us that support, even if in a different form.

CHAPTER THIRTEEN

THE PANDAS MONSTER

It was June 2013 and we'd planned our yearly getaway to the coastal town of Umhlanga, which is 20 km from Durban and a popular holiday destination for many South Africans. The summer climate there is humid and hot, but the June winter weather is pleasantly mild. We'd escape the dry and cold Johannesburg winter for seashells, sandcastles and the warm Indian Ocean.

David loved nothing better than going on holiday and had been looking forward to the trip for a very long time. He counted off the days on his calendar one by one, until finally the big day arrived. Unfortunately, just before we left he contracted a strep throat (streptococcal infection). For our family, going on holiday is never a simple exercise, owing to David's special diet and the number of nutrient supplements and medicines we have to lug along. Martin often questioned why I packed for any and every possible medical eventuality – and almost every time we went away ended up thanking me because without fail one of the kids would fall ill.

On a previous trip to Umhlanga we'd forgotten the Rehydrat, which is crucial when kids have repeated vomiting episodes. I remember Martin having to go to the Umhlanga Hospital in the early hours of the morning to beg for Rehydrat. He returned empty-handed as the hospital wouldn't give it to him without a prescription. Ever since, I have made sure our 'holiday mobile pharmacy' is fully stocked!

Soon after arriving in Umhlanga, we noticed that David had become irritable and unreasonable. The sudden onset and the magnitude of his

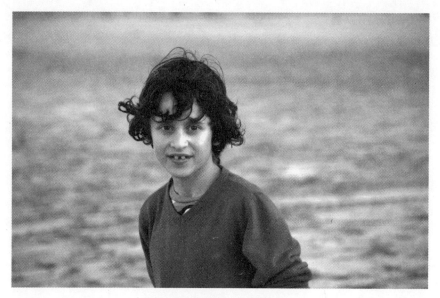

David on holiday at the coast

irrational behaviour was particularly scary and alarming. As the days passed these behaviours intensified so much that it became challenging to even leave our apartment. He became psychotic, and it was distressing to witness our son so deranged.

A 'simple' blood-pressure check

We decided to check David's blood pressure at Umhlanga Hospital as we thought it might be high and playing a role in his behaviour. However, taking his blood pressure proved to be quite traumatic. Nothing could prepare us for the trauma that followed. I went into the hospital to organise the blood-pressure test and Martin stayed outside with David in the parking lot, keeping him occupied until I gave the thumbs-up to come inside. Eli had stayed at the apartment to look after Aaron. The nurse was able to place the blood pressure cuff around David's arm without too much fuss. But as soon as she inflated it, he started to scream hysterically. At this point I didn't care much about what anyone thought of David's behaviour. All I wanted was to get an accurate blood-pressure reading. But this was impossible.

After numerous failed attempts, we left the hospital disheartened and concerned. It would have been one thing to have gone through all that pain and embarrassment and achieved results – but to walk away with nothing but a bruised heart felt unfair. It was just another blow to our weary beings as we tried to survive our so-called 'getaway' to Umhlanga.

Not such a good idea

The next morning, which was the Friday before Sabbath, we had to go to the supermarket to buy food. As we drove there in the car, we knew it was going to be difficult with David, yet I had insisted we do things together as I did not want us to be imprisoned by autism once again. I wasn't willing to entertain the possibility of Martin staying in the apartment with him while I went shopping alone. Part of the fun of being on holiday was to treat the kids and enjoy the excitement of spoiling them at the shops. I so badly wanted to experience the joy of being on holiday as a family that I was adamant we'd *all* go into the supermarket.

On arriving we decided to walk up and down the aisles as fast as we could, to avoid setting David off. As we turned the corner into aisle 4, we bumped into Martin's friend Gary, whom he hadn't seen for a very long time. David's anger had already been building since aisle 1. After giving Martin a big hug, Gary proceeded to get his body into a comfortable position for a nice, long catch-up chat. David, however, was having none of this. Reading the signs, Martin immediately told Gary that David wasn't feeling well and that he couldn't chat any longer. As can be expected, Gary thought Martin still had a couple of minutes just to say goodbye. When Martin insisted that he *really* needed to go immediately, we could clearly see that Gary felt uncomfortable and suspicious of Martin's apparently unfriendly demeanour.

Mere seconds later, David let out a huge scream. The kind of scream only a person being strangled to death can let out. In that instant, Gary realised why Martin wanted to cut his conversation short. The look on Gary's face will be etched in our memories forever: he'd probably never witnessed anything like it before. Without saying goodbye or uttering another word,

Martin simply marched David – still screaming at the top of his lungs – to the car park. This was a few floors and a three-minute walk away, and when you're in that kind of situation every step feels as if it's taking ten minutes instead of a few seconds. Time stands still and the whole experience is agonising and embarrassing.

We'd decided – before entering the supermarket – that if David had a meltdown I'd continue shopping while Martin walked David to the car. Upon eventually reaching the car, Martin placed David inside and stood outside watching through the window as his son went wild. David screamed and cried for a full 20 minutes without a single pause. We'd been through milder forms of these episodes throughout David's life but we'd never encountered such a breakdown before.

PANDAS rears its ugly head

Being in public places like a supermarket could cause David severe anxiety. He would try to block out the noise as the crowded supermarket became too overwhelming for him. Shopping in Umhlanga was even harder than normal for him as he had begun to restrict what he'd eat and would gag at the smell of certain foods. We didn't know it then, but this was a result of Paediatric Auto-immune Neuropsychiatric Disorder Associated with Streptococcal Infections (PANDAS), which would still take us a few days to discover.

His outbursts of uncontrollable rage were astonishing to witness. Suddenly, he would insist that all doors remain open. If we locked a door, he'd wake up in the middle of the night to unlock it. One evening in Umhlanga, I caught him unlocking the front door of our apartment and had to wrestle him to the ground to stop him going out. His irrational behaviour was escalating and we became quite desperate trying to figure out what had set this off.

Generally on the Sabbath, starting on Friday evening, we're meant to get dressed in our best clothes and enjoy a family meal after attending synagogue. David's day hadn't improved and we'd spent it trying to calm him down. His obsessive-compulsive behaviours worsened and he became dysfunctional. For us there was no getting dressed up, or planning the Sabbath meal, or attending synagogue together as a family. Quite the opposite – feeling scruffy and worn down by the events of the day, we decided to take him for a walk along the beachfront. This turned out to be a bad idea as we bumped into friends returning from synagogue along the way. Dressed to the nines, many were going to celebrate the Sabbath with family and friends over a warm, scrumptious meal. Some people wanted to stop and chat, but we 'rudely' brushed them off and continued walking. We knew that any break in our walk could trigger an explosion from David.

Eventually that evening, David fell asleep. On a Sabbath – when we switch ourselves off from telephones, television or other distractions – we usually enjoy peace and tranquillity. During these times, we normally spend hours discussing David's case and our next move. This time was no different.

A simple answer and an immediate solution

After chatting for a while that night, we came to the conclusion we couldn't carry on one more day with David in the state he was in. Although we don't normally speak on the telephone on Sabbath, I dialled Dr Jeff Bradstreet. 'I'm sorry to bother you on a Friday,' I told him, 'but I desperately need your help.'

Having listened to my pleas for help and my despairing description of the previous few days, Jeff was able to state with confidence that David was suffering from PANDAS. He said that one of the treatments for this condition was antibiotics and recommended Zithromax for David, which needed to be administered immediately. We hadn't given David an antibiotic since we had discovered his autism as we knew this could worsen his symptoms. Jeff explained that, in this case, we had no choice and needed to rescue David urgently.

I put down the phone and Martin and I quickly formulated a plan on how we were going to get Zithromax without a prescription at 11 pm on a Friday night in Umhlanga. As I'd already broken the Sabbath by speaking on the telephone, we decided it would be best for me to drive to a nearby pharmacy Martin suspected might be open. I wasn't a confident driver at the best of times, and having to drive at night to a place I'd never been to before rattled me. Martin reassured me and gave me accurate directions to the pharmacy. As I was leaving he tapped my shoulder, looked me in the eye and said, 'Don't come back without the medicine.'

I climbed into the car and started what felt like a really long journey. As the road twisted and turned, I remembered Martin telling me, 'When you think you've gone too far you need to carry on – because it's very far down the road, tucked away next to a petrol station.' I doubted myself as I followed the road on and on. I didn't have a GPS or Google Maps in those days, so relied on my instincts. It was dark and scary but I was determined to get there.

Eventually, I turned a corner and found the petrol station. When I saw the words 'Pharmacy' flashing in blue lights next to it, I breathed a huge sigh of relief. Half the battle had been finding the place. Sitting in the car, I collected my thoughts and planned how I'd convince the pharmacist to give me an antibiotic without a doctor's prescription. I jumped out, neatened the rags I was dressed in and, with a straight back, walked over to the pharmacist's counter inside.

I told the pharmacist: 'I'm not a drug addict; I'm just the mom of a child with autism who is really sick and needs an antibiotic called Zithromax. I'm begging you to give me only *one* Zithromax. I'll return tomorrow morning with a prescription from my doctor as I live in Johannesburg and need to make the arrangements for this – but I'm not leaving this pharmacy without a Zithromax.'

'Okay lady,' he casually replied. 'I don't mind – calm down. I'll give you three tablets and you can come back with the prescription in the morning.'

Holding onto the precious tablets and thanking him for the thousandth time, I left the pharmacy and jumped back into the car. When Martin opened the door of our holiday flat, I held the Zithromax aloft in triumph. We danced with joy and immediately went to David's bedroom. We woke him up and gave him the Zithromax. I had a glass of wine and went to bed.

Pulling David from the jaws of PANDAS

By the next morning David's symptoms had improved significantly and we knew the Zithromax was working. As the days passed he got better, but the moment we stopped the medicine his symptoms flared up again. When we returned to Johannesburg, we started a rigorous protocol of immune-modulation therapy. Little did we know then that we'd be fighting PANDAS for years to come …

Looking back, what is most terrifying is that, had we gone to a 'traditional' GP in Umhlanga, he or she would immediately have prescribed a psychiatric medication or referred us to a psychiatrist. Given David's symptoms, that would have been understandable. And, to develop this line of thought to a more-than-possible conclusion, David might have been admitted to a psychiatric institution from which he might never have been released.

Only someone thoroughly trained in autism would have recognised that David was presenting with the criteria for PANDAS. Doctors who understand autism will always check for strep titres in the blood as part of their biomedical treatment approach, as this is a common marker to be investigated when treating autism. Sadly, those who don't understand autism will see PANDAS as unexplained manic and psychotic behaviour.

Understanding PANS and PANDAS

Paediatric Acute-onset Neuropsychiatric Syndrome (PANS) is a clinical diagnosis given to children who have a dramatic – sometimes overnight – onset of neuropsychiatric symptoms, including obsessions and compulsions, and food restrictions. They are often diagnosed with Obsessive-Compulsive Disorder (OCD) or an eating disorder, but the sudden onset of the symptoms separates PANS from these other disorders. In addition, there may be symptoms of depression, irritability and anxiety, and difficulty with schoolwork. In most cases the cause of PANS is unknown, but is thought to be triggered by infections, metabolic disturbances and other inflammatory reactions.

Like those with PANS, children with PANDAS have an acute onset of neuropsychiatric symptoms, specifically obsessive-compulsive behaviours or tics (involuntary, purposeless movements). However, PANDAS patients test positive for a recent streptococcal infection, such as strep throat, peri-anal strep or scarlet fever. Like PANS patients, they may also suffer from uncontrollable emotions, irritability, anxiety and loss of academic ability and handwriting skills. People caring for the child may observe flapping.

If your child has been diagnosed as autistic, the possibility of both conditions being present should be investigated as soon as possible by a medical professional.

In both PANS and PANDAS, the symptoms occur as episodes and vary in severity over time. Numerous treatments are available to alleviate the symptoms experienced in the two conditions. Note, however, that each treatment requires careful direction from, and monitoring by, a medical team trained in the relevant field.

CHAPTER FOURTEEN

LOSING AARON

On returning home from the coast we continued David's treatment for PANDAS and he resumed his ABA programme at The Star Academy. Eli went back to school for the second half of Grade 3, having excelled academically in the first term. Aaron was developing on track as far as we could see, with no visible cause for concern. I went back to work and tried to close the chapter on the awful experience in Umhlanga. I felt I had been aged by our encounter with PANDAS; and had certainly become much wiser about the underlying causes of – and treatments for – autism.

Aaron's development, however, was always on my mind. I wished away time so he would get older and have a proper conversation with me, putting my mind at ease that he'd escaped the grasp of autism.

A bad decision

Aaron was 16 months old in September 2013. As he was suffering from recurrent ear infections, we decided that the best course of action would be to insert grommets to drain the fluid from his ears, thereby reducing the occurrence of future ear infections. I'd done my homework and covered what I thought were all the possible dangers or threats to Aaron's development. Considering that he was genetically vulnerable, I was trying my best to avoid any environmental triggers that might cause regression.

It never crossed my mind that an anaesthetic might be unsafe for Aaron. On the morning of the procedure to insert the grommets, the anaesthetist came past on her ward rounds before going into theatre. I asked her what anaesthetic she'd be using and she replied that nitrous oxide was safe for children; it was the method she used most often for her young patients. As she proceeded to speak to the patient in the bed beside us, it dawned on me that I should have checked on the safety of the anaesthetic. Not wanting to over-react, however, I dismissed the uneasy feeling I had in that moment and we proceeded to theatre. Something was telling me I'd regret this decision, but it is very easy to behave irrationally as a parent and I was trying to stay within the bounds of normality.

Over the months Aaron had already developed words and went into theatre as a 'normal' baby. The entire procedure took ten minutes and the Ear, Nose and Throat (ENT) specialist reported that he was happy with how it had gone. He'd successfully cleared the excess fluid build-up and inserted the grommets. Anxious for Aaron to wake up, I was relieved to hear him cry as he emerged from the anaesthetic. He was thirsty after the procedure and I handed him his bottle. Not suspecting that anything was wrong, I took him home.

As Eli got into the car when I fetched him from school that afternoon, he asked: 'Mom, why is Aaron not looking at me?' Aaron had not said his usual hello to Eli, and Eli immediately noticed Aaron's lack of eye contact. From that moment on, Aaron didn't speak again, losing all the words he'd previously used. He stopped waving goodbye and it was terrifying to see him run around in circles, spinning the wheels of his car, no longer playing appropriately as he'd done before with his toys. Within a matter of days after the procedure to insert the grommets we'd lost him, just as we'd lost David ten years earlier. I felt as though every bit of air around me had been sucked away, leaving me gasping and in pain as never before. It was gut-wrenching.

I'll never forget the fateful week when the lights went out for Aaron and I lost my 17-month-old baby to autism. But one thing I did know – this time around we had an army ready to go into battle for our boy ...

Confirming our darkest fears

John Galle, the CARD Affiliate Director, arrived in South Africa a week after we'd 'lost' Aaron. John was tall, with rosy cheeks, striking blue eyes and a raspy American accent. He had come to check on our programmes and, as usual, would be running our staff training. We confided our worst fears to him … that we suspected Aaron had autism. We also asked if he'd come around to the house the next day to observe our youngest child.

John was silent for a couple of moments, visibly shocked as he processed what we'd just told him. He'd been in South Africa not more than three months before, and Aaron then had clearly been developing on track. Knowing about our intense involvement with autism, John obviously suspected we might be over-analysing Aaron's development. But I knew in my heart that wasn't the case. We were in big trouble!

When John arrived at the house, Aaron hid behind Martin. He made eye contact and gave John a big smile. Martin and I then left John and Aaron playing on the floor in the playroom while we went to make supper, giving John time and space alone with our son.

An hour later, I went to check on them. We called Doreen in the United States and John told her what he'd noted: Aaron was not responding to environmental sounds, his language was noticeably delayed for a 17-month-old and he'd been spinning the wheels of his toy car instead of pushing it around the floor. Aaron wasn't pointing or following instructions any more, and appeared to be in his own world. There we had it … autism – our worst nightmare all over again. How could this be happening?

Doreen encouraged us. 'Martin,' she said, 'I know you're worried but you're going to recover this one. He's very young. Ilana, when you see him engaging in self-stimulatory behaviour, remember you're going to be doing everything possible to change that. Tell yourself it's temporary.'

I went to bed bewildered and in shock. I don't know how Martin and I got through the night. I sobbed so much I fell asleep exhausted, both physically and emotionally drained. Lying in the dark bedroom, I wondered when it was that autism had come to take my baby away from me. I'd been keeping watch over Aaron night and day. How had I missed autism when it had crept inside undetected and taken Aaron? The dull pain I felt followed me around for days. Martin was beside himself. This time I was the positive one, determined that Aaron would be fine now that we knew so much and had experts fighting in our corner. Martin was simply devastated – he could hardly speak he was so sad. That night, we both came face to face with the kind of pain that is totally impossible to describe.

Planning my next move

I sat down at my desk the day after John's visit and thought deeply about what to do. We'd been fighting for David for over ten years. Where on earth were we going to find the strength to fight autism a second time around when the first fight was still going on? Somehow, I found strength I never thought I had. Two things I was sure of – I needed to act very fast and I was going to fight to the bitter end. Reminding myself that I had ten years' research under my belt. I spoke to autism as if it were standing in the room beside me. I warned autism: 'Here I come – watch out!' I dug deep and started to plan my attack. Going straight to the cupboard, I found all the textbooks, notes and papers on biomedical intervention I'd collected over the years. I made appointments to speak to Dr Bradstreet; to Dr Kurt Woeller, an American biomedical doctor; and to a metabolic specialist and nutritionist in New York. I read the textbooks again from cover to cover, making notes for myself as I mapped out a plan to find a cure for Aaron's autism.

Starting ABA

In the meantime, we had to start ABA with Aaron. As John was in town, he designed Aaron's initial programme. My first question to John was: 'Do you think he'll ever talk again?'

His reply is imprinted in my mind forever: 'We're going to do everything in our power to make sure he does talk.' I drew a certain amount of comfort from John's reassurance.

John took advice from CARD's head office in Tarzana, United States, to make sure he'd made the best recommendations for Aaron. All the big shots agreed that we should follow Aaron's lead, and Natural Environment Training (NET) was recommended. Aaron was very young, and implementing child-driven therapy was the consensus for interventions at such an early age. The last thing they wanted to do was put him at a work table doing what we called Discrete Trial Training (DTT). John suggested I get together a team of only our top senior instructors, as we wanted only the best.

Over the next couple of days, I watched from my bedroom window as the team ran after Aaron in the garden following his lead. Aaron had lots of energy. We wanted to teach him the early social games of chase and peek-a-boo as targets in his ABA programme. It was quite a sight to watch the instructors running across the garden after Aaron.

Ten days on

It was a hot Johannesburg Saturday morning and I was sitting on the bench in my garden watching Aaron playing on the grass outside. This wasn't working, a voice screamed inside me. I was losing the fight. I'd seen absolutely no progress from Aaron since we started his programme ten days earlier. I followed my gut instinct and decided that NET was not the way to go. Monday came around and I instructed my team to start lessons in a DTT format but they refused, telling me they were obliged to follow the supervisor's recommendations. I was their boss but ethically the team wouldn't follow my suggestions, not wanting to upset the team of CARD supervisors remotely assigned to Aaron.

Firing the team

There was only one option open to me. To the utter dismay and shock of everyone concerned, I fired the entire team, including the two American CARD supervisors assigned to Aaron. I had phone calls and emails from team members cautioning me not to give up and to rethink my decision. However, I just knew there were too many seniors on my team and that this had been a mistake. Here were all these leaders, yet no one wanted to take responsibility as they were frightened to step on each other's toes. It was simply the wrong team dynamic. You can't have only seniors on a team. It has to be a mix of junior and senior instructors, and this is now very much part of our winning formula at The Star Academy.

At the time, I could only imagine what they were all saying about my decision: 'She has finally cracked and lost her mind.' 'Losing her baby has been the last straw.' 'It's an emotional decision and she's not thinking clearly.' I was certainly not giving up, but I wasn't going to waste another single day on a programme that wasn't working.

I knew that we had to start DTT with Aaron – that following his lead wasn't the correct decision. The team didn't want to go against the supervisor's recommendations, but *my baby's future was at stake*. My decision to fire the team took an enormous amount of guts on my part. At the same time, I didn't care about their feelings. What mattered was Aaron and only Aaron. I'd come up with a programme that would yield results.

By this time the news had spread to Doreen, and she called me to discuss my decision to fire the team. Doreen thought she had to convince me that ABA was the only route to take. 'What will you do if you don't do ABA?' she asked. I explained that I hadn't given up on ABA, and that my frustration was with the NET approach instead! Doreen understood immediately and I remember clearly what she said next: 'I always train my supervisors to listen to the parent and consider what they want. After all, the parent knows their child best. I apologise that they didn't listen to you.' We talked it over and decided to change the team, continuing with Peter Faraq, a CARD supervisor who'd been flying to South Africa regularly to devise programmes for some of the children at The Star Academy. I've taken Doreen's advice to heart, and at the Academy we listen to every parent if they doubt a member of their child's team for even a moment.

To the moon and back
I gave the orders to change Aaron's team; and selected three new instructors who'd remain on the new team for a very long time to come. I thought it over carefully. I wanted a team who'd go to the moon and back to ensure

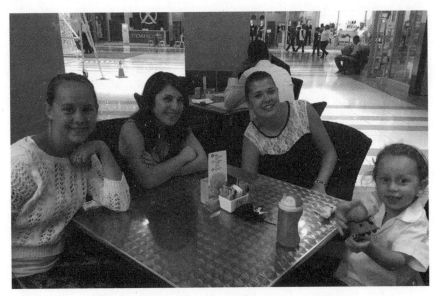

Aaron and his team (from left): Kirsten, Iana and Jacky

his progress, caring *only* about what would be in his best interests. I had no time for agendas or egos. I wanted a team who'd think of Aaron's programme before falling asleep at night and first thing when they woke up in the morning. It would be demanding working for me, and so I wanted a team who could go the extra mile. Today, that is something I expect from every Star Academy instructor.

JACKY VICENTE

I was looking for instructors who had energy, fire and tenacity. Jacky Vicente came to mind. She'd worked for The Star Academy for a year and had left to take a gap year in Portugal. She'd been back in South Africa working for us for only a few months. What I liked about Jacky was that she wasn't afraid of anything. I sent her a message to call me. She was sitting in church when she received my message and thought she was in trouble. Concerned about why I needed to speak to her, she stepped out to call me. I said: 'Jacky, I've lost Aaron and need to rescue him from autism – will you help me?' Relieved, she excitedly accepted my offer to join Aaron's team.

From the first moment she walked through my door to take her first session with Aaron, I knew I'd made the right decision. As much as Aaron was going to go through therapy I was going to be there, right by his side every step of the way, which meant I had to be comfortable with my team. Jacky's energy lit up the room and I trusted her instinctively.

BIANCA CASSINGENA

Bianca was next on my list. She'd taken me aside a few days back and asked to be on Aaron's team. By chance a space had become available. 'You know my speciality is babies,' she reminded me. 'Put me on the team – I can do this!' I was encouraged by her confidence and enthusiasm. Bianca and Aaron came to share a special bond and she was instrumental in his progress in those early days. Her firm yet caring nature worked well with him. A special chemistry between child and instructor is something that's considered essential at The Star Academy.

If anyone could get Aaron to imitate, it was Bianca. What I loved most about her was that she saw the glass half full and not half empty. For instance, if a child is learning to kick a ball using a physical prompt, Bianca will hold their hand so they'll instinctively know to use their foot. This immediately gives the child confidence. But what makes her particularly effective, not just for the child but for the parents, is her positive feedback where she tells parents: 'Look at how your child is learning to kick the ball – in another few days they're going to be doing this on their own' instead of, 'They still can't kick the ball on their own.' We believe in the children and their ability to learn through positive reinforcement. This isn't just our belief – it's evidence-based fact.

Bianca's positive outlook carried me through. She'd focus on what Aaron *could* do and build on this. She was mature beyond her years and an angel sent to carry my family through some of the darkest days of our lives. Today we have lots of angels at The Star Academy.

PETER FARAG

Peter had worked for CARD in the United States for over ten years. I'd heard rumours he was Doreen's blue-eyed boy, and he had recently qualified as a clinical supervisor, which allowed him to design and manage cases. When Peter stood next to Aaron it reminded me of 'Jack and the Beanstalk' as Peter was a giant and Aaron tiny in comparison. Peter would lift Aaron in the air, holding him above his shoulders and twirling him around. We started with our first workshop and Peter was probing to see how many gross motor imitation skills Aaron possessed. Imitation is key to language and a big focus.

Aaron was sitting in his high chair. Peter took two identical rattles and gave Aaron one. 'Do this,' he instructed Aaron as he shook the rattle. He waited for Aaron to pick his up and copy him, but Aaron didn't respond. Within a second, Peter took Aaron's hand and guided him to shake the rattle.

'Hey Peter,' I yelled – 'can't you get a baby to shake a rattle? They told me you were good?'

Peter looked at me and accepted my challenge. 'Watch and learn,' he spat back at me.

Determined to prove me wrong, Peter continued to try to get Aaron to shake the rattle. He sat opposite Aaron at the table. He tried on the floor, the couch, outside and in different rooms with different rattles. Aaron wouldn't shake the rattle. What was frustrating for me to watch was that Aaron had done this before – effortlessly. But that was before the anaesthetic had changed his life.

Now Aaron was refusing to do something as simple as shaking a rattle.

Peter asked me: 'What does he love? I don't want something he likes. Find me something he loves the most.'

Finding the magic key

ABA 101: A child will give their best response for the highest reward. Aaron's success hinged on us finding Aaron's highest motivator. At the time, the movie *The Lorax* was Aaron's favourite and I turned it on for him to watch. Peter waited patiently for Aaron to get lost in the movie. At just the right moment, he pushed 'Pause'. Aaron was moaning and wanted Peter to turn the movie back on. Peter delivered the instruction again: 'Do this', firmly instructing Aaron to copy him. What happened next was incredible. Aaron picked up the rattle and shook it as Peter had asked him to do, then flung the rattle across the room in a fit of rage. 'Thought I couldn't get a baby to shake a rattle?' Peter scoffed at me. We were so relieved. We'd found what made Aaron tick and would use movies for months to come to motivate Aaron to learn.

Unlike David, Aaron didn't cry and scream or kick up a fight. He was receptive to the ABA programme from the very outset. There I was, once again, sitting in a room going through ABA targets with my baby, who before autism set in was in perfect health, but who was now pale and visibly unwell. I didn't have time to be sad. I focused on the goals and turned them upside down so Aaron would be successful. I'd walk into the sessions and tell the girls that they'd get a turn with Aaron and I'd get a turn with Aaron. If the target was to bang a drum, we'd work together to get Aaron to bang the drum. I'll never forget sitting on the floor beside Jacky working through the gross motor imitation targets as one by one we ticked them off the list.

Slow but positive steps

Aaron had to learn how to blow. I bought every whistle imaginable. Despite the array of whistles, toys and gadgets around them the team couldn't get Aaron to blow. I was determined he'd blow. Blowing was important for speech. I demonstrated for Aaron while the team stood back and watched me. I blew so much I became dizzy and short of breath. I kept delivering the instruction for Aaron to blow, keeping him engaged and ensuring he didn't become frustrated. When Aaron let out a breath of air, I fell to the floor exhausted. The team clapped and cheered for him. Aaron was doing relatively well. His progress was steady. We needed to move faster but we were certainly gaining ground.

Today, when I watch him blow out his birthday candles, I'm overcome with emotion and gratitude. Most parents don't even think about an act as simple as this. For parents of autistic kids, however, this is a major achievement.

Those long months of silence

Aaron didn't utter a single sound or word for five months. From 17 months to 22 months, he was completely silent. Other babies of the same age would be building their language, burbling out new words daily. His development had come to an abrupt standstill. It was terrifying. The weeks went by and I remember pushing him in his red pram, going for a walk with Martin as we usually did every Saturday morning. We walked down the road in silence. Aaron's future and ours was uncertain and it was upsetting to be confronted with the fact that he wasn't talking – at all. How would we cope with two children who weren't able to speak? It was unimaginable and we were numb. There were no emotions left.

Prayer and a light for hope

On one particular Saturday morning we decided to go to synagogue in the hope that it would force us to stop wallowing in self-pity. I'd been crying for most of the morning and arrived with swollen eyes, my hair a mess and my clothes hanging on me as I'd again hardly eaten anything over the previous few months. We were sitting on chairs in the shade of a tree watching Aaron play on the jungle gym, when Simone Hope walked over to us. Simone's daughter Naomi was working for me at The Star Academy as my personal assistant. We had started to chat about Naomi when Simone blurted out: 'What's wrong with you? You look terrible!' I broke down and told her about Aaron, that he'd stopped talking and how we'd started an ABA programme for him.

Simone had advice on a way out of the situation we found ourselves in. It was related to an ancient mystical Jewish text called the 'Perek Shira', which believers recite daily for 40 days as a spiritual remedy to overcome troubles. It is customary to light a candle to burn continuously for the 40 days and 40 nights during which the text is read. The candle is a physical act of bringing G-d's spirituality into the home. By reciting the sections of 'Perek Shira', I'd be tapping into the spiritual world, opening a channel for my prayers to be answered. I figured I had nothing to lose by following Simone's suggestion.

Drained from a typical day which included managing two ABA pro-grammes, for David and Aaron, being there for Eli and managing The Star Academy, I sat down at the dining room table. It was already 11 pm but I forced myself to open the prayer book. I read the prayers one by one, tak-ing them in and focusing on my spiritual connection to G-d. One of the prayers in the book touched my heart in particular. There was a picture of a swallow perched on a wooden branch and the prayer read: 'So that my soul shall praise you and shall not be silent, G-d my Lord, I shall give thanks to you forever.'

I started to believe that my prayers could change our fate. Simone had cautioned that if the candle went out for whatever reason, it wouldn't be a good sign. The candle needed to burn continuously. I watched over the can-dle, worrying that something might happen to extinguish the flame. Aaron's candle never went out and it burnt brightly for 40 days and 40 nights.

Turning Aaron's voice back on

At a conference I attended in the United States, I had met a metabolic specialist. When Aaron went silent, she seemed the right person to call for answers. We were desperately searching for a magic button to turn his voice back on. The specialist was a respected scientist in her own field and well known in the field of autism. We spoke for over two hours to get to the bottom of the sequence of events that had plunged Aaron into autism. The specialist led me through a scientific maze as she explained the meth-ylation cycle; and I realised that the anaesthetic (nitrous oxide) Aaron had received when the ENT inserted his grommets had derailed his methyla-tion cycle. In addition, the nitrous oxide had caused inflammation in his brain, which in turn had resulted in the breakage of the wiring in his brain. She prescribed folate as a treatment for Aaron, and directed me towards published research on the use of folate supplementation in addressing a dysfunctional methylation pathway.

I read the research, which indicated that children with autism might be suffering from cerebral folate deficiency and advocated supplementa-tion with folate to alleviate the symptoms of autism. I immediately put this information to the test by buying a bottle of folate. Would something as simple as this make the difference I'd hoped for?

A miracle?

Within 48 hours of starting folate, Aaron's voice returned and he said '*buh*'. It came unexpectedly. I was chatting with Jacky, and the next thing Aaron started to say '*buh, buh, buh*'. For the past seven months, we hadn't heard a sound from Aaron. I looked at Jacky and she looked at me and started to cry – the tears were rolling down her face. Had we heard correctly? We stood frozen, praying we'd hear him say it again, and he did. Finally, a flicker of hope! Never had I been so happy to hear Aaron say '*buh*'.

Reflecting on the previous few days, I realised that I'd started the prayers, the candle and the folate at the same time. So was it the folate or the prayers? I can confidently say it was a combination of both. Adding the spiritual dimension to the physical treatments was crucial. I was only meant to keep the candle burning for 40 days and I was only meant to say 'Perek Shira' for 40 days. It's been over three years now, and there's always a candle burning in my house and I don't miss a day of saying this prayer. In addition to this, today my prayers are filled with thanks to G-d for giving me back my boy and answering my prayers. The light of the candle guided Aaron out of the darkness and into the light.

Setting up Aaron's language programme

Since we'd established The Star Academy, we'd enrolled a PROMPT instructor from New York who travelled to South Africa three to four times a year to train our instructors in this approach and programme. And each time we brought a trained speech pathologist and PROMPT instructor to South Africa, I'd host and train a group of South African speech therapists, as well as our instructors at The Star Academy, in PROMPT. My vision was to entrench the PROMPT methodology in South Africa for future children who would need it.

The PROMPT instructor from the States had diagnosed Aaron with sensory-processing disorder and severe apraxia. When she observed Aaron for the first time at 17 months, she told my team that his targets for the next six months were to be 'oh', 'ah' and 'm'. I knew we'd never recover Aaron with progress that slow and with such small expectations! The instructor, of course, had set Aaron's goals based on how he was presenting at that time. My team will not forget the fateful day on which she broke the news to me that she had only small expectations for Aaron in the months to come. I calmly told her there was no way in hell I'd accept those three targets or her expectations for Aaron. He was going to do better than that for sure!

We began to argue and my team didn't know where to hide. In my innermost being I knew I was going to find a way. Each expert I was consulting added a piece to Aaron's treatment programme but I could envisage the whole picture. ABA, PROMPT and biomedical intervention combined would weave the magic we were looking for. She could only see one piece of the puzzle.

A potential setback

I was sitting on the floor next to Bianca and she was working on Aaron's language targets, which now included what we called echoics. We'd say a sound and Aaron had to echo back the sound he'd heard. We were working on getting the sound *buh* under control. Even though Aaron could randomly say *buh*, he needed to say it back to us when we asked him to. That's how we'd get it under control. He was making good progress, but what I noticed when he echoed *buh* back to Bianca was that he was using only one side of his mouth. He looked like a stroke patient. In that moment Bianca caught my gaze and knew at once what I was thinking. 'Ilana,' she said, 'stay calm. I saw what you saw; he'll start using the other side of his mouth soon.' Although worried, I remained hopeful.

In the end, although it would take three years, we overcame apraxia! This is quite a victory considering how severe Aaron's apraxia was. Very few people get this type of result.

If you, the reader, are wondering what we did right, perhaps the answer lies in the word 'intensity'. In most cases, the parents of children diagnosed with autism are advised to do speech therapy for 30 minutes twice a week. With Aaron, we did oral motor exercises and PROMPT every 30 minutes for seven hours a day. He would have his naps and a break, and we'd start again. Add to this his biomedical protocol, proper nutrition and a toxin-free environment, and you have a winning formula.

In our experience at The Star Academy, only one child in a hundred will come right on ABA alone. You need a combination of one-on-one intervention and the other things just mentioned to get a measurable result.

Many parents bring their children to us looking for a quick fix. But as good as ABA is – and of course it does significantly contribute to a child's progress – what's needed in terms of re-establishing language acquisition is total commitment.

Our very own 'Dr House'

Dr Bradstreet was our own version of Dr House of television fame. He started Aaron on medication to support his immune system and ordered tests so we could ascertain what was causing his autism symptoms. The lab tests confirmed he had yeast and bacterial overgrowth which contributed to his hyperactivity, so we immediately put him on courses of oral Nystatin and Vancomycin. We scheduled a weekly call so we could keep a check on his medical protocol. Dr Bradstreet knew how important it was to act fast. The longer Aaron was under attack from environmental insults and the longer it took us to put out the fire, the less chance we had of recovering him. Aaron responded well to the treatments for yeast and bacterial overgrowth and became much less hyperactive. He also started to slowly break through the world that encapsulated him and kept him from us.

I was very afraid to check Aaron's results for Landau Kleffner Syndrome Variant (LKSV). This was a blood test done through Dr Anne Connolly, from Washington University's neuromuscular division. Some children on the autism spectrum had been testing positive for LKSV and this meant they had ruptures in the capillaries in their brains' blood vessels. We'd done this test for David at five years of age and he'd tested positive. I knew this test was an indicator of prognosis and was even afraid to suggest it to Dr Bradstreet, but I did. Dr Bradstreet encouraged me to conduct the test for Aaron. 'Don't be afraid,' he told me. 'Once you know what you're dealing with you can start treatments to reverse or correct it.' A week later the test kit arrived and we drew blood to send to Dr Connolly. When the test results were released and emailed to me, I was petrified to open them. I peeped at the results and had never been so happy to see the word 'negative' emblazoned on a piece of paper in front of me. I was dancing from relief. This was a very good sign.

Kick-starting Aaron's engine: Judy's high-dose omega

Once Aaron started to get his sounds back, we called Judy Chinitz, to ask how she felt about putting Aaron on a high dose of omega. Her response was optimistic. She explained that Aaron's development was like a car that had stalled, and that a high dose of omega for a couple of weeks might act as jump-start cables. Within 48 hours of Aaron taking the omega, his eye contact returned and he began to produce more sounds. This was good news for us, as it indicated the presence of a brain inflammation that could be treated. We had been there before. We reported the results of the high-dose omega to Dr Bradstreet, and he organised a test at a French lab to check Aaron's inflammatory markers.

We were taking steps in the right direction, and slowly but surely building Aaron's medical-treatment protocol. Treating autism is not a sprint – it's a marathon. It requires trial, error and endurance.

Working it out with Dr Woeller[8]

Dr Woeller had always been a sensible doctor and I'd relied on his advice for David many times over the years. Dr McCandless had recommended him, which was a feather in his cap. His understanding of biochemistry

---

8 For more information on Dr Kurt Woeller and on biomedical autism treatment resources for parents and caregivers with loved ones on the autism spectrum, visit www.autismrecoverysystem.com.

and the underlying causes of autism was extensive. The call I made was very intense: I demanded answers from him, pressing him for direction. Dr Woeller explained the role of brain inflammation, directing me to the 'Stop Calling it Autism' (SCIA) protocol that had been endorsed by a number of medical doctors in the United States.[9]

The high-dose omega had been a clue, which we used as a building block going forward. Further treatment entailed the anti-inflammatory ibuprofen and high-dose probiotics to line the stomach (ibuprofen can be really harsh on the stomach lining). The SCIA protocol made sense to me and I immediately started Aaron on rounds of ibuprofen.

We saw an overall improvement in Aaron from this anti-inflammatory treatment. He became calmer, more aware of his surroundings and started to follow our instructions. It became easier for him to produce sounds too. Dr Woeller explained that ibuprofen would help to put out the fire in his brain.

Dr Woeller's four pillars of autism treatment

Dr Woeller's four pillars in treating autism cannot be faulted. They are:
1. –Dietary intervention
2. –Support in the form of biochemical supplements
3. –Assessing the digestive system for chronic infections and treating those
4. –Methylation

We'd tested Aaron's inflammatory markers both at Great Plains Laboratory in the United States and at a French laboratory, and both tests concluded that he had high inflammation markers. We'd need to treat the inflammation while at the same time uncovering its cause. Without a doubt, the anaesthetic he'd had for his grommets had played a role in setting his brain on fire. I read the SCIA protocol over and over and over. We had a window of opportunity, that was true, but this window was also closing a little as each day passed.

---

9 Visit www.stopcallingitautism.org for more information on the protocol.

BRAVE CHOICES

With a life sentence of autism hanging over us, Martin and I were often faced with difficult dilemmas that required brave decisions. We had to attack autism aggressively in the hope of defeating it. Determined to outsmart the disease this time around, we leapt time and time again to save Aaron. Knowing at the back of our minds that every treatment had a side effect and that none was risk-free, we grappled with every decision we took. Of course, we would only allow ourselves to take very informed decisions, which meant that we had to do our research every step of the way; and to weigh up the relative advantages and dangers of Aaron's treatment options.

Whether or not to start certain treatments with our sons had already become an obstacle for us when it came to David. 'What if the ibuprofen damages David's stomach lining?' 'What if this medication harms his liver?' These thoughts often prevented us from agreeing on trying out certain treatments.

At another level, Martin and I realised that we had very few choices in such matters since David was already seriously ill. As each day passed, the chances of our firstborn becoming fully verbal became less and less. I didn't want Martin to blame me if something went wrong.

Over time, however, we learnt to debate each issue fruitfully. We didn't always agree, but we certainly always managed to find a workable solution.

CHAPTER FIFTEEN

SURVIVING DAVID'S TEENAGE YEARS

Over the next few years, not only were we dealing with an angry teenager with autism but we were also in the fight of our lives to save Aaron. Whenever we thought things were settling and getting a little better, we were surprised anew by the overwhelming heartache of autism and its strength in pulling us down. The next few years were gruelling: the autism battle raged on like a wild fire, consuming us with its heat and intensity. We needed every ounce of our strength to fight back. It took grit to wake up in the morning and get through another day. We had to hold it together and constantly make the choice to be strong. Eli needed us and so did The Star Academy. It would have been easy to just give up, but there was too much at stake. Martin fought alongside me every step of the way, holding me up as we waged our battle together.

A typical day consisted of managing two ABA programmes, one for David and one for Aaron, raising Eli and fitting everything else in between.

Giving new meaning to the 'terrible teens'

David's teenage years were particularly challenging and demanding, and he regularly tested our faith and endurance. Gut-wrenching reports about behaviours David engaged in or things he couldn't do became a regular part of our day. We were stripped of so much as parents, while also becoming increasingly exposed to horrific details of David's violent outbursts and descriptive accounts of his self-injurious behaviour. When we thought things couldn't get worse, they did …

His daily report might describe how many times he'd hit himself, screamed or tried to wring his nose, the last a common behaviour he'd developed to show his disapproval or anger over something he'd been asked to do.

David even had a punching bag, which was placed on the floor in his station at The Star Academy so his team could redirect him to hitting the bag instead of himself or them. This was needed especially when his behaviour was automatic, which meant we couldn't stop it and had to find a better way for him to channel this behaviour.

The cycle of self-inflicting pain begins

David began to hit his head repetitively as a little boy. I remember feeling somehow grateful that he never tried to hit, bite or attack his instructors. But this changed as he became a teen. As if it wasn't bad enough to hear about how he had tried to hurt himself, we had to face that he had started turning on his team, lashing out at them and having to be restrained.

I have to say that what we were exposed to as parents was inconceivable. It was a living hell. I'm not afraid of much after living through the long days that turned into years of David's tantrums and bad behaviour. David's Behaviour-Intervention Plan (BIP) was regularly updated and tweaked as the supervisors allocated to him by CARD over the years scrambled to remain on top of his case.

His daily report, painstakingly put together, verified how many times he rocked, toe-walked, flapped his hands or struggled to make a sound or copy a word. Over the years I got used to what felt like endless lists upon lists of skills David struggled with or couldn't achieve. Each time we tried to find a way to teach him, he'd master the skill but wouldn't maintain what he'd learnt, regressing time and time again, losing everything and knocking us back to a point of zero progress. On top of that, the opportunities David had for learning were in any case few, as he was unstable most days.

Being subjected to David's aggression and self-injurious behaviour is not what I'd signed up for when I became a parent. If I'd taken a glimpse into the future and seen what our life would become when I held that little baby in my arms for the first time, I'm quite sure I'd have had a heart attack on the spot.

We got used to carrying around an emoji cushion so that on days when his frustration and sheer anger was sky-high, he could hit the pillow and not his head or nose, which were often bruised and blue from his attacks on himself. His behaviour was automatic a great deal of the time. On a good day, there would be only one or two incidents.

Behaviour management 24/7

Because David's entire programme was centred on behaviour management and simply preventing him from hurting himself, his learning was put on hold for a long time. We tried all the tricks in the book to get him to calm down. David was angry most of the time and appeared uncomfortable in his own skin. Driving with David became a scary experience and I used to worry he would knock his head straight through the glass window, which was something he threatened to do on numerous occasions. Breakfast was the worst time of the day: he refused to eat, repeatedly hitting his head and screaming as he hit the table or himself.

The days of behaviour management rolled into weeks and the weeks into months, then years. I'm eternally grateful to my Star Academy team who managed his behaviour so well during those dark days and supported us through it. We were only really at peace when David was asleep. I'll never forget waking up to his screams and the sound of him hitting his head against his bedroom wall in the morning. I'd shake myself awake from a deep sleep to the sound of the loud thuds coming from his room. What a way to start the day!

We felt robbed of all those normal things parents experience when raising a child. Conversations in my kitchen revolved around solutions to David's anger instead of soccer or cricket matches or the other normal things parents raising a typical child are privileged to discuss. Our pain and anger were deep and mostly we just tried to survive. It felt like there would be no end to the torture we were exposed to every day.

Nothing is more painful for a parent than to witness their child unhappy or in pain. As my ABA team studied his behaviour graphs and regularly updated or changed the BIP, Martin and I looked for medical answers. We spent hours consulting doctors on how to calm David down and restore his gut health and overall well-being. As parents we refused to accept that we would be subjected to this painful life of witnessing our child beat himself up forever.

Being viewed as a bad parent

Going out to the shops or anywhere in public became impossible. Aaron was only two years old at the time, and if David burst into a fit of rage Aaron would start screaming from sheer fright. Eli would just stand there staring in front of him and wishing he belonged to a different family. Standing in line at the grocery store was particularly tough. As there are no lines in Pick 'n Pay or Woolworths for special-needs kids, I often stood in the senior citizens' line. This evoked countless comments from old people, some of whom tapped me on the shoulder to tell me to move to another queue. I'd be nervous standing in that line, as I was anticipating an old lady hitting me on the head with a handbag at any moment and was regularly subjected to much vocal criticism for having dared to stand there.

One day, when an old lady tapped me on the shoulder asking me how I dared to stand in the senior citizens' line, I explained that my son had autism and could become impatient. She didn't believe me and told me I was being very cheeky. Looking over at David, I could see his anger and impatience building. I told her that in ten seconds my son would demonstrate why I was standing in that line. She continued to badger me, until David belted out a scream while at the same time hitting his head. A scared Aaron also started screaming. By now, the entire store was fixing its gaze on us. I felt a thousand eyes burning into the back of my neck but continued to stare straight ahead, not daring to look around. But more was to come.

Eventually, when I did look up, I caught sight of the familiar face of an acquaintance in the line next to ours. Her head was tilted to the side in pity and her eyes burning with deep concern for me as she asked me in a gentle voice whether everything was 'okay'. I wanted to scream at her that everything was clearly not okay. Did it look like I was okay? As David continued to dish out punches to himself, I courageously asked her whether *she* was okay. She quickly reverted to unpacking her shopping basket.

As I left the store, I wished the earth would open up and swallow us. I looked forward to crawling into bed that night, pulling the duvet over my head and enjoying the silence, alone in the safety of my bedroom where I'd be away from the world for just a few moments.

This is just one example of what we went through during that dark period when David's aggression and tantrums were out of control. We had many more incidents when David 'lost it'. I used to consider carrying a water gun to spray him with during these meltdowns, but was advised against it by my ABA team (they felt shock at my suggestion). I fantasised about darting him like a game ranger darts a wild animal and wished I had a tranquilliser injection I could carry around in my handbag to use on days when his tantrums and anger were extreme.

The terrible teens: if only …

Living through David's teenage years presented many moments of sadness and, of course, endless challenges. My hopes and dreams for my son often evaporated into the atmosphere, as if they'd never even existed at all. One such time was when my niece, born a month after David, called me excitedly to say goodbye as she'd been packing to go on youth camp for three weeks. I envied her parents, who'd have the house all to themselves for the duration of camp. I couldn't even imagine what it would be like to be free for three weeks. What would I do? Where would I go? But David would never be going to youth camp. There would be no discussions around which trunk or suitcase he'd be taking with him, no running around the shops for things he'd need, excitedly getting his clothes ready or buying camping equipment. There would be no goodbyes at the airport or photographs of David spending time with his friends at camp.

When my next-door neighbour's son hosted a year-end disco for his Grade 8 class at home, I sneaked a look over the wall. I saw teenagers dressed in jeans and the latest trendy T-shirts chatting, laughing and dancing to the music. They seemed so innocent and carefree as they enjoyed the opportunity to experience life, make friends and live their dreams. David had no chance. He was clinging to life shackled to the chains of autism, under my supervision and care 24 hours a day, seven days a week.

All these moments along the way were hurtful. Yet we'd consider what we'd lost for only brief moments, and then move on: there was no time to wallow in the pain and sorrow that life had dealt us.

Mom: Enemy number one

Of everyone around him, David was most angry with me. I was the person telling him what to do day in and day out. Get up, get dressed, eat breakfast, hurry up, let's go, let's go … He'd wake up in a foul mood and often tried to headbutt or threaten me by tilting his head to the side as I walked past him preparing his breakfast or packing his snacks and lunch tin for school. He'd try to headbutt his team too, and even his father, when Martin held him to stop him injuring himself.

I was desperate and, as much as I'd been trained on how to manage his behaviour, as a parent in that moment I'd forget everything I'd learnt. Staying calm and collected became very tricky when he screamed for the one hundredth time that day or tried to headbutt me once again. My patience was wearing down fast.

At that time I was also managing Aaron's ABA programme and searching for medical answers to secure his development. What we went through then is beyond description. It got to the point where I even wished that David would die. To witness your child so unhappy and so angry and dysfunctional for so long got to me and I'd tell Martin that it would be better if our son died. I saw no point to his life apart from our torture. Which parent would want to live through days of hearing their teenage son cry like a one-year-old and scream like a wild boar? Nothing we did to help him or to try to turn this around worked. Worst of all, Dr Bradstreet had passed away and we no longer had him to fall back on.

Desperate times mean desperate measures

At this point there was very little we wouldn't do to try and stop David's violent outbursts. From Zoloft, which didn't help at all, through Risperdal to medical marijuana, we tried it all. We were put in touch with a marijuana dealer from Durban who had a reputation for having the right blends and could put together a specific remedy for David. Medical marijuana had become a common treatment in America and I joined a parents' Facebook group called Charlotte's Web, where parents shared their stories of using medical marijuana to treat epileptic seizures, autism and other illnesses. I remember meeting the connection from Durban in the parking lot at the Pick 'n Pay centre. He opened his boot and gave me the marijuana for David while I slipped the cash into his pocket. I had visions of being arrested but didn't care as we desperately needed to find a solution for David. But even the marijuana wasn't enough to stop his rage.

David struggled to fall and stay asleep. He couldn't eat or speak, and screamed or engaged in self-injurious behaviour for most of the day. He picked the skin on his fingers until his hands bled, and would pick any scab off his body until there was a visible hole in his flesh. He was destructive and miserable and we were broken parents. Afraid of what the future might hold, we struggled to keep our heads above water.

I finally crack

I'll never forget the day in the kitchen when David finally pushed me too far. This time it escalated so quickly that, before I had realised what I was doing, I found my hands around his neck. As I squeezed tight, I suddenly let go. David looked as if he was passing out and about to drop to the floor. The room started to swim around me as I thought I'd killed him. Thankfully, he came to. I started screaming and screaming and couldn't stop for hours. I had to take a tranquilliser to calm down and I vowed I'd never put myself in such a position again. When in future he screamed or tried to headbutt me, I simply walked out the kitchen or sent him to his room until he calmed down.

Martin's reactions were the opposite of mine. When David had his violent episodes of headbutting and hitting, he'd hug him and hold him and try to calmly talk him through it. David would headbutt him a few times, but Martin managed to stay calm. He would tell me that he felt so sorry for David as he was only a child; and that we had to find a solution to the underlying medical cause for his fits of rage.

No safe place

Going to the ocean had always been one of David's favourite things to do, and he relished every moment we'd allow him to swim and float in the waves. But in those teenage days, even in the water where he was doing the very thing he loved most, he'd scream and shout and beat himself up, causing quite the scene for onlookers.

It was quite normal to see David running down our corridor from the kitchen to his bedroom, hopping along in anger, crying and shrieking. It looked as if a bee had stung him and he was running away from the pain. We doubled the dose of Zoloft but that didn't work at all.

We'd cry on Doreen's shoulder, confiding in her that David was having these terrible meltdowns. She did everything in her power to help us, which was something we always admired about her. Doreen suggested we make contact with an American doctor who'd had years of experience treating autistic children medically. Doreen made the introduction and the doctor replied. She had a year's waiting list and undertook to visit South Africa 12 months later …

CHAPTER SIXTEEN

AARON'S RESCUE OPERATION

I combed through every detail of Aaron's and David's ABA programmes daily. There wasn't a lesson I was unaware of, or didn't know how to implement myself. I understood why the lesson was there and I made sure we were moving forward.

At this stage our pace for Aaron was steady and we focused on keeping him motivated. He enjoyed his sessions, which remained scheduled for seven hours every day. I had teams of people coming in and out of my house for both children. Sometimes I had two instructors with Aaron at the same time, one being in training. I could have employed a bellboy just to open and close the gate to my house.

We had weekly workshops during which the team members would get together and watch each other work with Aaron. When we did PROMPT, we made sure everyone knew how to prompt and was delivering the prompts in exactly the same way. They'd practise on each other, leaving no room for error. David's team met regularly to discuss behaviour management and how to keep his programme moving forward. We had to work through his behaviour, never giving up on teaching him skills acquisition.

One of the most important issues I identified early on was that effective team communication would be critical to success. There was so much detail – and ensuring that everyone was on the same page was crucial. I set up a WhatsApp group for both Aaron and David, and the teams reported back to me after every single session. The report would highlight any aspects the other team members should take note of, so that by the time they started their next session they were clear as to where their focus had to be.

Aaron's ABA-specific programme contained a list of lessons and goals for him to master, but I decided that weekly goals would propel his progress forward. We'd set five goals each week that the team had to make sure were covered in each session. I was confident this would be a game-changer, and it was. If we were struggling with anything, the team would take a short video clip of the lesson and post it on the group for feedback. That way we could ensure that everyone was being consistent and pick up any problems. The WhatsApp feedback made all the difference and we began setting weekly goals for David too.

Mickey Mouse or Donald Duck

Our Star Academy team members all had different strengths, based on the experience they'd gained working with the children assigned to them over the years. Quincy Jansen had been working for me for just over two years and he'd built a reputation for being an exceptionally smart and capable problem-solver who always came up with solutions. He was particularly well versed in PROMPT, and had impressed our PROMPT trainer from New York many times with his natural ability and talent.

Quincy had been born and raised in a town in the Free State called Welkom, and came from very humble beginnings. He'd heard about The Star Academy from a friend and working with special-needs children appealed to him. Quincy was really talented and I involved him, drawing on my skilled staff for particular expertise depending on what Aaron's programme dictated at any particular point in time. Quincy would come in daily to prompt Aaron and train my team in PROMPT.

We'd just started teaching Aaron object labels, which is an important language lesson aimed at building language content. Aaron would need to know hundreds of labels such as 'chair', 'book', 'train', 'teddy bear' and so on, so he could draw from his language bank when he wanted to request something or when the time came for him to have a conversation. This can be very tricky and requires a child to use a number of skills to be successful. We'd been struggling with this for a few days and thus decided to lean on Quincy's problem-solving skills.

Quincy identified the piece of the puzzle we'd missed: Aaron wasn't tuning in to the instruction. Quincy's solution, which worked well, was behaviour momentum. This entails running through a few quick mastered targets with the child to tune them in before delivering a new instruction for them to follow. Making sure he had eye contact with Aaron, Quincy told him to 'touch nose, touch head, touch tummy'. Aaron followed Quincy's commands, listening to the instructions given. It's an art to get a child to tune in and then grab the exact moment to deliver a new instruction the child hasn't yet mastered. We were all watching, holding our breath. Quincy delivered the instruction for Aaron to pick up the Mickey Mouse figurine in front of him. This meant that Aaron had to listen to the instruction, scan the field in front of him that consisted of Mickey Mouse, Donald Duck and Pluto, select Mickey and hand it to Quincy.

I'd had weeks and weeks of David screaming through this lesson years earlier and what I was thinking and going through in that very moment was agonising. I waited and watched as Aaron carefully selected Mickey and handed it to Quincy. We cheered so loudly the next-door neighbours could hear us. We followed through with some more trials to satisfy ourselves that Aaron could discriminate. Thankfully, if we got him to tune in and used behavioural momentum, he'd always be successful in selecting the correct item. Over time, of course, we'd fade our prompts. Quincy had managed to unlock this lesson for Aaron, and it would be the gateway to teaching him other important language lessons to come.

Tragedy strikes

Quincy was only 27 years old. He entered an IRONMAN race, collapsed as a result of a heart attack and was rushed to hospital. The doctors fought to save him as we all waited next to the phone until late that night for news that he'd made it through. The news wasn't good and Quincy died, leaving behind the girlfriend who'd been the love of his life. We were all simply devastated. It was difficult to comprehend that someone so talented and young would have their life cut short so unexpectedly. He was making a real difference in the world and had been instrumental in changing the lives of many autistic children for the better. We all tried to come to terms with the fact that Quincy's mission in life was done.

The next day I met with his mom, who'd come to Johannesburg to fetch his body for burial. She was going to take him back home but stopped past The Star Academy to meet us. I had a large lump in my throat. Dressed in traditional black clothing, she sat hunched over on the couch outside my office. We brought the children that Quincy had worked with to meet her one by one, introducing them and explaining to her the wonderful work he'd done and how he'd contributed to each one of them. Quincy will never be forgotten by his colleagues and his memory lives on in the children whose lives he touched.

My secret weapon

Bianca, who was leading Aaron's programme, was accepted into a Master's programme in educational psychology. She and Aaron shared something special. Only the best candidates made it to the short list of successful applicants and I was ecstatic for Bianca. At the same time, I was sad for Aaron as she'd played an important role in his life and our ABA journey had just begun.

As much as we loved Bianca, however, I'd been around long enough to know that no one is indispensable. Parents often become worried about team changes or on hearing the news that one of their instructors is leaving. But as long as there's a pool of instructors to draw from, the programme will survive the change and the child will continue to make progress.

We had a strong pool of instructors at The Star Academy and I started to do some homework and investigation to decide on the best replacement for Bianca. Rumour had it that Iana Tchoukanska, who was working at our Pretoria Academy, had a couple of years of ABA experience and was the most suitable person to take over from Bianca. Iana was also studying towards her Board Certified Behaviour Analyst (BCBA) degree and had a reputation for being extremely hard working.

I didn't waste any time and called her to discuss the possibility of her spending three days a week in Johannesburg working with Aaron. It would mean an hour's drive each way, depending on traffic. Very often the morning traffic from Pretoria to Johannesburg was very congested and unless Iana left her house at 5.30 am, which she'd often do, she'd be stuck in traffic for more than two hours. I suggested she initially take on the position for six months and then decide if she wanted to continue. Iana not only agreed to take over from Bianca but also continued to lead and manage Aaron's programme for the next three years. She was unconditionally dedicated to Aaron's success. Originally from Bulgaria, she was tenacious and very professional. She became known as my secret weapon; and her contribution to Aaron's ABA programme ended up being immense.

Peter supervised Aaron's programme for six months. We'd been checking in with Doreen, and she decided to move the case to Carolynn Bredyck from the San Juan Capistrano office of CARD. Both David and Aaron would be under her supervision for the next couple of years.

The rarest diamond of all – Carolynn Bredyck

Carolynn, a Board Certified Behaviour Analyst and Senior Clinician at CARD, had the experience and expertise to ensure our success. Not only would she be there to try and help David manage his anger and frustration, but she would also be responsible for directing Aaron's programme.

It's not usual to have the privilege of working with, and having your children's cases supervised by someone such as Carolynn. Her clinical expertise was in another league and changed our lives forever. Her role was truly instrumental in helping us make it through autism. Moreover, I trusted Carolynn instinctively from the very moment we were introduced to her, and her empathy carried me through an extremely dark period in my life.

Carolynn wouldn't travel to South Africa in person, but for over four years she Skyped in and directed Aaron's and David's programmes remotely from America. Iana, in charge of Aaron's programme on the ground, would follow her direction; and so would Ashleigh, who was managing David's case locally. We spoke to Carolynn for at least two hours every week without fail. The years of mentorship Iana and Ashleigh received from Carolynn would filter down to the other children at The Star Academy for years to come.

Carolynn was one step ahead and knew what was coming next. We'd send her short video clips of both kids and she'd work from those. It's one thing to programme for a child you see weekly or even monthly in person, but Carolynn managed to pull it off, perfectly setting goals remotely and without observing David or Aaron in person. That in itself speaks volumes. She paid attention to detail and was always up to date with the latest developments, logging daily onto the online programme containing David's and Aaron's latest ABA data. She'd write notes for the teams to find in the morning, leaving them instructions on a particular lesson or intervention. And would always come up with solutions when our deliberations about the best ways of achieving our goals failed to get anywhere.

She was also the only CARD supervisor who could successfully deal with me. Carolynn was always able to say the right thing at the right time and pick me up when I needed lifting. There were many times when Aaron would get stuck on a lesson or not make the desired progress, which was extremely worrying for me. Carolynn managed to put things in perspective and gave me confidence that we were on the right track. Having three children of her own, she understood what it meant to be a mom. She never set unrealistic goals *and* she set the correct pace.

Somehow, we crept into her heart.

Aaron's second birthday, 30 May 2014

It was Aaron's second birthday. I kept his birthday low-key and bought a small round chocolate cake with candles to mark the day. I was happy he could blow out his candles. I didn't pause too long or I wouldn't have made it through the day. Aaron was making fair progress. He was learning to pronounce different consonants and vowels and even a few blends (this is where words are first broken down into vowels, consonants and syllables then put back together again to form whole words). Just like David, he was paving the way for other children with autism who'd need help in future.

We used PROMPT a great deal to teach Aaron to 'motor plan' the different sounds. Every letter of the alphabet he mastered was a conquest, and I didn't rest until I found a way for him to reach the point where he was able to say a particular sound.

Progress!

By two years and three months, we were in a much better place than we'd been a few months before. Aaron's receptive language had come a long way and he'd already learnt a good number of labels, easily discriminating between objects he knew and new ones we introduced. His attention, eye contact and overall awareness had improved in leaps and bounds. However, he still wasn't learning from his natural environment and wasn't talking. His play skills were still significantly delayed for his age.

Carolynn explained he'd need to learn different play sequences that would impact on his language and, later, his ability to establish and maintain friendships. For example, he needed to push the train on the tracks and stop at the station for people to climb on. He'd need to push his car around the track, wash and paint the car, and come up with different ways to play with the car. These early skills would be important for him and would be the building blocks to doing comprehension and essays at school.

Namenda: a game-changer

We'd planned to speak to Dr Bradstreet at 11 pm SA time. This particular call was pivotal for Aaron. It was winter in Johannesburg and I'd crawled into bed exhausted from the day. I'd fallen asleep when Martin shook me awake for the call. 'Dr Jeff – you need to make it easier for Aaron to speak,' I insisted. 'It's still too hard for him.' There was a long silence. 'Are you still there?' I asked. He was thinking it over. What he recommended next was a miracle drug for Aaron. Namenda, a medication originally used for Alzheimer's patients, was now a treatment used to help children with autism. He'd recommended it for David many years before, but we hadn't been brave enough then to try it as we were worried about possible side effects. I'd already had more than a sneak preview into what life could be with a child who couldn't speak! This time I dived straight in when it came to treatments.

Dr Bradstreet recalled the story of one of his patients – a young boy from Germany who'd taken Namenda for 18 months only from the age of three years and had gone on to shed his diagnosis of autism.

The plan was to give this medicine to Aaron for a period of time only. Once we bridged his apraxia, we'd wean him off it. Aaron responded within the first three days and we witnessed an immediate improvement in his vocals. Over the coming weeks, it would become easier and easier for Aaron to form the sounds. He was beating his apraxia. In no time, he started to copy words. I can only describe hearing each new word as being like tasting a drop of purest honey dripping from a honey jar.

I can't express the relief and joy we experienced. It was exhilarating, and the grey cloud looming over Aaron started to lift.[10]

Carolynn also introduced Kaufman cards, a speech tool designed specifically for children with speech apraxia. They were a highly effective tool in helping Aaron become more vocal. The several different approximations of a word on the back of a card allowed Aaron to *always* be successful and he gradually learnt the sounds, syllables and words. We had a number of Kaufman cards as targets in his lesson programmes for a full year. Aaron had to practise the word over and over until he succeeded in pronouncing it.

Play, play, play

I turned my cottage into a dream playroom for Aaron with every toy imaginable. I must say I enjoyed shopping for all the toys; and spent my free time surfing Amazon looking for toys that would teach him different play sequences. Carolynn gave us an idea that helped Aaron learn play skills. We'd tape ourselves playing with a toy car or train and then play it

---

10 Investigating the need to regulate glutamate in the brain is an important consideration to discuss with your doctor when deciding on your child's treatment protocol. Preliminary information can be found at https://www.ncbi.nlm.nih.gov/pmc/articles/PMC4141213/, accessed 11 April 2019.

back to Aaron for him to imitate. Video modelling worked well and Aaron learnt the play sequences in no time. We cherished the progress he made, celebrating every target met along the way. Eli was highly reinforcing for Aaron, and I'd use him many times to model play sequences for his little brother.

We relished every moment Aaron would play and engage with his toys. As his play skills strengthened, we moved on to more complicated sequences including pirate ships, Paw Patrol rescues and Mickey Mouse Clubhouse. It was important for Aaron to learn all of those, and he did.

CHAPTER SEVENTEEN

DAVID'S SEIZURES: A NEVER-ENDING NIGHTMARE

We couldn't predict that our life was about to change forever on that fateful day in July 2014 – one that seemed no different from any other when it started at the crack of dawn, with David waking up at 5 am. I got out of bed as I did every day and got the kids dressed and ready for school. It was to be a normal work-filled day and I'd mapped out my time at the office, which included juggling Aaron's ABA programme with several meetings.

The office was up the road from my house – two minutes' drive away. I'd rushed home to pop in and check on Aaron when my phone rang. I saw the name of one of David's instructors flashing on the screen. 'Come now! Come quickly! David's had a fit; he's blue in the face, and lying on the ground; we think he had a seizure!'

Time stood still. As I flung myself in the car and sped up the hill to David all I could think of was a friend who'd recently died from a fatal seizure. Fortunately, I didn't have too far to drive. I almost stopped breathing as I drove up the hill. When I got to The Star Academy I flew out the car and ran to the playground, where several of our instructors were huddled around David, who was lying in his vomit, unconscious and seemingly barely alive.

'Does he have a pulse?' I screamed.

'Very faint.'

'Did you call the ambulance?' I heard myself asking.

'They're coming.'

'Call them again!' I yelled back.

I lifted David in my arms to take him inside, as he'd been lying outside on the wet grass. He continued to throw up and I had no way of knowing whether he'd lost functioning or skills. I remember trying to stay as calm as possible and suppressing my concerns. After what seemed like an eternity, the paramedics arrived. They asked me a few questions and I told them David had autism. By now David's vital signs were good. I asked them to stop the nausea, but they couldn't: he might have a reaction to the anti-nausea medication. I was aware of every minute of his nausea, as he couldn't stop throwing up.

I kept asking the paramedics questions, but they firmly asked me to step aside and let them do their job. 'No! I won't step aside!' I hissed. 'He's on a special medical protocol and I have to know exactly what you're doing and what's going on.' One medical mistake could have knocked us back ten years! I received a stiff glare but ignored it. I called Martin.

'David's okay, but we're going to the hospital.'

'Oh! Did he fall out of a tree?' Martin asked.

'No, he had a seizure ...'

'A seizure!'

The paramedics were loading David onto the stretcher when I told them that we weren't going anywhere until I'd spoken to my doctor. I called him to ask which hospital would be best equipped to deal with David and his advice was to go to the hospital where my paediatrician was based.

It was my first experience in an ambulance and I hoped it would be the last. It all seemed so surreal. Martin was waiting for us as we arrived at the hospital and they wheeled David into Casualty. It was only then that David started to focus again. I placed his iPad in his hand and asked him a few questions:

'David, how old are you?'

'Twelve years old,' the iPad replied.

'Where do you live?'

'Johannesburg.'

Pointing to Martin: 'Who is this?'

'Martin.'

A once-off incident?

David's first seizure had come as a huge shock as it had been completely unexpected. We nevertheless sighed in relief, knowing he hadn't lost any functioning or skills. David fell asleep and we were admitted to the paediatric ward where we waited for two hours for our paediatrician to grace us with his presence. When he finally arrived, his advice was to take David home and observe him over the next 48 hours.

When we got home, David ate a big meal and spent the rest of the afternoon on his bicycle as if nothing had happened. That night I checked on him every hour to make sure he was breathing. We hoped it had been just a once-off seizure. Because I hadn't been there when it happened, it was easy to block out the experience and we carried on with life as normal, as if the seizure was going to be just another story to tell.

Reality kicks in

Eight weeks later, I witnessed David having another seizure. I'd been in meetings the entire morning and had just arrived home. As I walked through the door, I noticed David sitting at the dining room table with his back to the front door. I found it strange that he didn't turn around to acknowledge me as he usually did, and an uneasy feeling settled over me. At that moment David's arms went up in the air and became stiff; his head turned to the side and he started shaking. I ran to him screaming, trying to stay calm. I lay him down on the floor as his body jerked from the seizure, but the worst part was that his lips and fingertips turned blue and his eyes rolled back. I turned him on his side and began CPR.

My mother-in-law was visiting and I shouted at her to call an ambulance. She panicked, froze and just stood there screaming. David was blue, shaking, and it appeared to me that he wasn't breathing. I really thought he had died. The only thing I could think of was to drive him to my doctor. As I picked him up to take him to the car, I tripped and fell over him. This was a hideous feeling. Fortunately, his recovery had started; his body stopped shaking and the fall that had lifted his shirt showed his naked stomach moving faintly up and down. 'You're alive!' I screamed – 'You're alive!'

My mother-in-law finally called the ambulance. She held the phone to my ear and the person on the other side gave me instructions. He asked me to check whether David had a pulse. Initially, I couldn't find one. But as the time went by, his breathing became stronger and I could see his tummy moving up and down faster. I was worried about the loss of oxygen and, once again, the possible loss of *skills*.

A second major diagnosis for David

David started vomiting just as the ambulance arrived. The paramedics gave him oxygen, checked his vitals (which were normal) and sped off to the hospital with David and me. The Casualty doctor phoned the paediatrician, who officially diagnosed David with epilepsy. The paediatrician ordered a prescription for Epilim, but Dr Bradstreet preferred Keppra and we followed his advice.

Still in the Casualty room, I passed David his iPad and asked him a few questions.

'David, what is Mom's cell phone number?'

'O83 xxxxxxx,' he correctly typed out on his keyboard.

'What's your brother's name?'

'Eli,' the iPad spoke for him. His responses showed once again that he hadn't lost any skills.

The onset of David's seizures may have been a result of rapid brain changes as he approached puberty, combined with the underlying causes of his autism, including inflammation of the brain. Even though the seizure looked very bad, we tried to see the positive in what had happened. If David had been having invisible sub-clinical seizures before, it was now evident that his brain at times had irregular activity. We hoped that putting him on anti-epileptic drugs would bring about the *real* improvement we'd hoped for all these years. Sadly, that wasn't the case at all.

* * *

It was now official. David had autism *and* epilepsy. This was a lethal mix

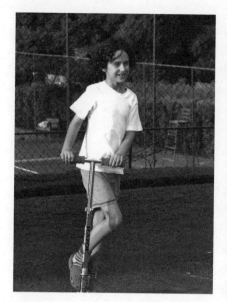 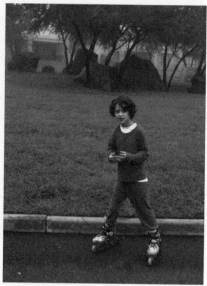

David's various adventures

of diagnoses that sent me into a spiral of depression. Wasn't it enough that David had autism?

I became anxious that David would have a seizure and die. If his team were a couple of minutes late in dropping him back from an outing, I became so panicked I couldn't breathe. I'd think the worst; imagining they were late because he'd had a fatal seizure. I still feel like this most days, and our life has never quite been the same since seizures entered it and changed it forever.

Checking in: our daily reality

Every Friday, David goes on the Gautrain accompanied by his The Star Academy instructor to spend the day in Pretoria. Fridays are stressful, and the team will check in with me regularly. Below example of my WhatsApp check-in from the team:

8.30 am: Leaving for train station
9 am: Arrived at Rosebank Station
9.15 am: Just boarded the train

9.55 am: Arrived safely at Centurion Station

10.30 am: We're at rock-climbing

11.30 am: On our way to bike-riding

12.00 pm: Safely at bike-riding

13.00 pm: On our way to train station

13.30 pm: Just boarded the train back to Rosebank

14.10 pm: Arrived at Rosebank Station and on way to the car

The drive from Rosebank Station to my house takes 15 minutes – sometimes 20. I'll hover near the CCTV screen waiting for the car to arrive with David. If they're a few minutes late, I become so worried I can't think straight. I'm always waiting for *that* phone call. The only time I get to be at peace is when I'm sleeping. I can never be away from my phone. Let me explain why.

One day, David went home early from school as he didn't look well. When I got there later, I called Martin to discuss which medical treatment I should administer. These types of issues happen often and we always consult each other to determine the best course of action. That day I'd covered all the bases, and wanted to spend some time observing Aaron in the cottage at my house to check on his ABA programme. I couldn't do this with David at home so I called my mom to ask if David could go over to her home for an hour. She of course agreed, and I dropped David and Eli there.

By the time I got home my mobile phone's battery had died. I left it charging in my bedroom while I went down to the cottage to be with Aaron. I'd been watching his session for 20 minutes when Aaron's instructor's phone rang. She picked it up as it was a strange number. I could see on her face that something was very wrong. 'It's Eli – go now, hurry, David has had a very bad seizure.' The room started swimming around me. I was walking to my car as fast as my feet would carry me but it felt as if everything was in slow motion. I grabbed my mobile phone on the way and saw that I had ten missed calls from my mother, from Eli, from Martin and from my office. It was crazy to think that, in the 20 minutes my phone had been charging, so much had happened.

I drove to my mother's house dialling Martin's number, but he wasn't answering. I eventually got through to my mom, who told me tearfully that David's seizure had been really bad and had gone on for a very long time. 'Mom, focus!' I yelled at her. 'How long did it last?'

'Ten minutes at least,' came the reply. I almost drove into the car in front of me.

'Mom, think carefully: Did it *feel* like ten minutes, or was it really ten minutes, or are you not sure? Did you time it?'

She hesitated. 'I can't be sure – maybe it was five minutes,' she finally said.

'Can you be sure it was five minutes or was it three minutes?'

'I don't know,' she replied. 'Just come.' She put the phone down.

While I'd been speaking to her, Martin had been trying to call me on the other line. I called him back and he too was on his way to my mother's house. When my mom couldn't get hold of me, she'd called Martin at his office. She was hysterical on the phone, crying and telling him that David was dead. Martin said that, although he was concerned, he was pretty sure she'd been overreacting. He tried to explain to her that people may look dead when they go into the recovery state after a seizure, and that it was unlikely that David was really dead. Had she taken his pulse? She hadn't taken a pulse and Martin told me how at that point she'd put the phone down. He ran out the office but the lift wasn't coming fast enough, so he took the stairs to get to his car. When he got to the bottom of the staircase the door was stuck and wouldn't open. He kicked it repeatedly to get it open and sped off.

I arrived at my mom's apartment building and parked my car as fast as I could, taking the stairs rather than waiting for the lift, running as fast as my feet could carry me to the third floor. As long as I live, I'll never forget the scene when I entered the bedroom and saw David lying on the bed. He was surrounded by eight paramedics. One of them took me aside and said: 'Your son who had the seizure is fine. His vitals are fine, his oxygen-saturation levels are fine; he's sleeping now. But your other son is *not* fine – he's in the lounge shaking and in a terrible state … I think you should come with me now.'

Eli's traumatising experience

When I walked into the lounge, Eli was sobbing. He looked at me and said: 'I thought he was dead.' I'd trained Eli to lay David on his side, and to time the seizure and call the ambulance. He had done all those things, but when David had wanted to sit up to vomit, as happens so often with nauseous epileptic patients after a seizure, Eli had followed the instructions I'd given him to the letter and pushed his brother back down. Eli was feeling as if he'd placed David in danger, and was so distressed he was shaking like a leaf.

The paramedics left and, an hour later, David woke up as if nothing had happened. He got dressed and we walked him to the car. Again, he hadn't regressed in any way. We, however, had aged a couple of lifetimes.

Encountering partial seizures

David attends gymnastics daily, and it has become a significant part of his life.

On a particular day, he'd gone with his instructor to gymnastics as normal. He'd jumped on the trampoline and they were walking to the bars when suddenly David fell forward. He lay on the ground pale, motionless,

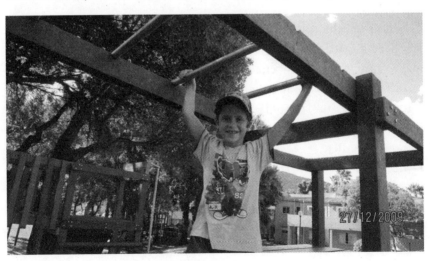

A young David at gymnastics

his unresponsive eyes wide open. After a few minutes he started to regain function but was weak and couldn't walk unassisted. I was in a meeting when my assistant called me out, asking me to contact David's instructor urgently. I dialled her number nervously. When I got through, she said: 'David's okay, but I'm not sure whether or not he's had a seizure.' She explained what had happened, and said she would send me a picture she'd taken of David after he'd fallen forward so I could see what I thought. While I was speaking with her, I immediately walked to my car and started driving to the gym. When I received the picture on my phone and looked at it, my heart missed a couple of beats.

That picture will be forever imprinted in my mind. Looking down at the lifeless image she'd sent me, I drove as fast as I could to get to him. Luckily, when I arrived, he'd already regained most of his functioning but was still very pale. I sensed he was oxygen deprived, drove him home and instinctively put an oxygen mask on his face.

On the way home I called Martin and we decided to watch David for half an hour before deciding on the next step. Once again Martin raced home from work and we watched over David who, by now, had responded well to the oxygen mask. We could gradually see the colour return to his face and satisfied ourselves he didn't need an ambulance or immediate medical care.

I discussed the episode with his neurologist, who established that this had been a 'partial' seizure. We were used to seeing David have a grand mal seizure, so was this better or worse? In some ways, I felt that partial seizures were almost worse than grand mal seizures. When he was having a grand mal seizure, I could see his body shaking. I'd also become used to understanding that this was a seizure. Making sense of a partial seizure was much harder.

The seizures haven't stopped and they range in severity from mild to incredibly frightening. They can happen anywhere and at any time, and this does nothing to help our stress levels. A recent flight saw David being wheeled off a plane in an ambulance after he had a seizure as we landed. Needless to say, I'm now nervous to fly anywhere with him.

Still looking for solutions

David has taken medication to control seizures for many years and is still reliant on this today. We're working on getting to the bottom of why he even needs it and hope the future will bring a solution. Finding a paediatric neurologist prepared to look for answers in South Africa has been extremely challenging. The focus was on David's autism, and the conclusion drawn was that children with autism can have seizures. There was no motivation to look *beyond* autism for possible causes of epilepsy. But *why* should a child with autism seize? Inflammation in the brain, maybe? This caused me, once again, to look abroad for help.

We still have long conversations with our paediatrician in New York on possible ways ahead. The epilepsy medication doesn't treat the cause: all it does is prevent the seizure. A thorough investigation into the real causes is necessary. Working with our United States doctor to solve this issue has been comforting.

While the epilepsy medication reduced the frequency of David's seizures, his explosive rage was unpredictable for a very long time. I learnt only years later that the specific medication he was taking was known to induce rage. When we finally moved to a different treatment, we noted a significant reduction in his anger and irritability. No doubt the old epilepsy medication, on top of the occasional PANDAS flare-ups, had added to his irrational behaviour.

A long time after David's first seizure, I met an adult with epilepsy and was able to ask her a number of questions about how she felt when she had a seizure. Although her description left me shocked and made me feel terribly sad for David, I couldn't pull myself away from the conversation. She described feelings of depression, dizziness, regular nausea and wanting to commit suicide … I just had to find out as much as possible, because all this time David hadn't been able to tell us accurately how he'd been feeling.

CHAPTER EIGHTEEN

AARON SOARS HIGHER AND HIGHER

I don't really know how I got through the early days of Aaron's ABA pro-gramme. But the adrenaline kicked in and I just kept going. Every single day required my full commitment as I kept both ABA programmes on track. I made it a rule that my team for Aaron had to be completely differ-ent from David's team. I wouldn't allow a team member to work with both kids, as that would have weighed too heavily on them. ABA instructors take upon themselves an enormous responsibility, and hold the future of the child they are working with in their hands.

Being the boss at work didn't make things any easier.

Aaron was now three years old and one-and-a-half years into his ABA programme. His health had improved dramatically. His apraxia was fad-ing away. Most of the medications and supplements we were using for him worked instantly. We were managing to treat his derailed methyla-tion cycle successfully with folate and B12; and to reduce significantly the inflammation in his brain by rotating a number of anti-inflammatories on a weekly basis. The immune support we gave him extended the time inter-vals between his treatments for the yeast and bacterial overgrowth in his gut. We were also getting a handle on how to regulate glutamate in his brain. All of this translated into measurable results. One of them was that Aaron experienced a clear burst in his acquisition of skills.

Luckily, our amazing son Eli had remained well. Martin had taken over the responsibility for his schoolwork and other school activities, but our middle child was low maintenance and needed very little from us. He excelled academically and was a very easy and confident learner.

The importance of effective communication

In four years, I never missed a day reading over Aaron's WhatsApp feedback from my team. My role was to motivate them and ensure effective communication and consistency. Entrusting your child's future to someone else is never easy. Parents of children going through ABA will tell you that this is one of the hardest things to deal with. As much as I had insecurities and wanted to do it all myself, I could never be Aaron's primary educator and certainly wouldn't be physically capable of doing seven hours a day with him. Finding a balance between interfering in the way lessons were delivered and entrusting team members with the space to do their job wasn't easy. Luckily, Aaron never cried, screamed or fought with his team. He found them highly reinforcing and was happy for the interaction. This was very different from my experience with David, who fought and screamed for days and weeks on end.

There was no better feeling than receiving a message that Aaron had mastered a target or said a new sound or word. These small victories kept me sane and encouraged me to push forward.

Every minute of every session with Aaron was important for his recovery. This meant that my team had to pay attention to detail *all* the time. They had to read the WhatsApp feedback from every session every day, and had to be very sure about how they were implementing Aaron's programme. There was no room for error.

In my heart I knew what needed to be done and wasn't going to lose this momentum. It wasn't an option. Calm came over me as I focused on the daily targets. I didn't miss a single detail and when the afternoon shift arrived to take over from the morning instructor, I'd make sure to brief them thoroughly. I'd relay the important achievements of the morning session and what goals they needed to focus on; what Aaron was struggling with and what they needed to achieve in their session. I was not going to let the pit of autism swallow our precious baby and poured all my energy into his programme. Each day I'd put on my bullet-proof vest while burying my emotions deep inside.

The detailed expertise needed to conquer autism is enormous. But although the mission is fragile and tricky, it *is* possible.

It's all in the detail

When I sat down to write this section of the book, I contemplated for days on how to put into words the details and lessons we followed for Aaron, as there was just too much to tell and I didn't know how I'd squeeze four years of work into a few typed pages.

One word of caution here: just because one child grasps a language-acquisition concept in a certain way does not mean that all other children will get there in the same way. *Every child with autism is different and will learn differently from others and in their own time.*

MAKING EYE CONTACT

Carolynn was not to be negotiated with when it came to teaching Aaron eye contact. She stressed the importance of it over and over again. It is also one of the most basic requirements for social interaction. Without full eye contact, Aaron would miss important information.

At the beginning we'd try to get at least a glance from Aaron, building this up slowly until he could hold eye contact for three to five seconds and then longer.

Eventually, what worked with Aaron was video modelling. We'd record me, Martin, Eli and the entire instructional team responding to their names with both eye contact and the vocal follow up. Then we'd prime Aaron with these videos. He picked up on what we were showing him in no time.

As his fluency in vocal speech improved, we also increased the eye-contact requirements, until eventually he was looking at us 80 per cent of the time.

Aaron began pulling on my face so I would look directly at him when he spoke to me, demanding my eye contact and attention. This felt like an enormous achievement. For parents of typically-developing children, this can sometimes feel annoying. For us, it was pure joy.

BEING ABLE TO POINT

The ability to point is one of the prerequisite skills in language acquisition.

Aaron was struggling to form a point with his left hand. This meant doing different strengthening exercises (fine-motor strengthening) every two-and-a-half hours. It was three months before Aaron could point his finger independently.

ORAL MOTOR SKILLS (MOUTH, JAW, TONGUE AND LIP EXERCISES)
Aaron's oral motor skills were underdeveloped and not working properly. We had to focus on activities to strengthen and develop his mouth, tongue and lip movements. Working on Aaron's oral motor skills would be crucial in ensuring his speech production.

At any given time, Aaron had multiple targets in his programme. We practised them every half an hour on the hour, seven hours a day. Aaron struggled to stick his tongue out and we practised this over and over again. A very young baby is normally able to imitate this gesture without much effort. We brainstormed about getting Aaron to stick out his tongue, trying everything we could think of. Even puckering his lips was difficult for him, and we placed a special plastic jar with a hole in it over his mouth to teach him how to do this. We stimulated Aaron's facial muscles through frequent massage and used something called the 'Z-Vibe' to strengthen his tongue muscles and ensure that he could lift his tongue up and around in his mouth in order to talk clearly.

At around 18 months (when autism started), Aaron lost the motor skills he'd previously had for proper chewing. Feeding became challenging as he simply didn't know how to chew any more. Even swallowing was an issue. We had to re-teach all these skills. Day by day and through the multiple interventions and positive reinforcement of his team, he learnt how to chew again. He'd drool a lot and we'd get him to swallow every 15 minutes by running our hands under his chin and offering him regular sips of water. Aaron also couldn't suck from a straw and that was yet another mountain he had to climb during his recovery.

Today, he eats all kinds of food. He even prefers water to juice, and fruit to sweets. Like any other kid, he has his preferences. He sips from his water bottle effortlessly, as if there has never been a problem. When we watch him drink with a straw now, we forget about the previous battles. And we all melt as he generously dishes out butterfly kisses with a perfectly rounded pucker ...

Just shows what ABA can do.

MATCHING

One of the early language skills for a child is to be able to match similar objects. Aaron couldn't do this and we tried many different ways to get him to learn this skill. Determined to get him to master it, we practised on the table, on the floor and on the bed, and even placed the items in separate boxes mounted on the wall. Short of standing on my head, I ensured that we tried every single variation of matching. I thought about matching at 2 am in the morning and drove my team crazy until, a few days into this lesson, Aaron finally mastered the skill.

Once he realised what was expected of him and when the reinforcer we used was sufficient as a reward, Aaron matched beautifully, requiring no prompts. He mastered the skill within days of starting his ABA programme.

We relished each accomplishment along the way. We'd have to work hard to achieve them, often breaking down solid walls to reach our goals. If our targets weren't reached within a few days, I'd call meeting upon meeting of my team members to get them to crack the code that would lead to success.

NON-VOCAL IMITATION

Imitation is one of the early prerequisite skills to vocal language, and Aaron would need to master a long list of non-vocal imitation targets to form the foundation of his imitation skills as we worked towards getting him to vocalise. We'd had a taste of what life with a non-vocal child could be like and were well aware of the work and effort it would take to turn fate around.

For example, it proved to be a struggle to get Aaron to jump. Jumping normally emerges between the ages of two-and-a-half and three years. Finally, Aaron lifted himself off the ground with both feet and was able to jump. Years later, the feeling I experience when I see my little boy jump on a jumping castle at birthday parties is priceless. 'Come Mom, jump with me on the rocket ship,' he asked me at a birthday party. We held hands, and as I jumped up and down with him on the red and green jumping castle my heart was filled with gratitude. Something as simple as jumping is not something our family takes for granted.

ECHOICS: A MASSIVE BREAKTHROUGH

Our aim was to get Aaron to first echo back consonants, vowels and blends of consonants and vowels. We worked our way through the list of age-appropriate sounds one by one. The mastery of each sound was a massive accomplishment. Knowing which sounds to work on – based on the order in which they emerge in a typically-developing child – was helpful to us in setting Aaron's goals.

It was all very systematic and aimed at guiding Aaron through the stages of language development he'd missed out on. In the afternoons I'd join my team in the cottage while we worked on single sounds. Carolynn recommended an interactive app on the iPad, called SpeechStickers. Each time Aaron pressed the character he'd chosen to speak, it would repeat the consonant or vowel in exactly the same way and he'd have to imitate the sound. When he got to the end of the exercise, he'd be rewarded with popping balloons and cheers from the characters in the app. SpeechStickers was a silver bullet and helped Aaron gain better control over his vocals.

Finally, Aaron started imitating words and our careful laying of the foundation in the weeks building up to this started to pay off. PROMPT was one of the main interventions to help Aaron overcome his apraxia. To hold a conversation Aaron needed not only the ability to form sounds and words, but also a rich language bank that he could draw from.

PLAY SKILLS

Aaron's play skills were non-existent at the beginning of our ABA journey. Teaching him these would play a major role in his future ability to navigate the social world and was also critical to language development. In order to teach him play skills, we began to take him through the different stages of play, which unfolded as his skills developed. We made a list of all the different play skills Aaron needed; and ticked them off one by one as he grasped the fundamental concepts of the different kinds of play. Aaron's play skills evolved and, after careful programming and direction from Carolynn, he was able to play in ways that were appropriate to his age.

Today Aaron can play for hours on end. He loves nothing better than to stay in his pyjamas on a Saturday and play with all his toys. His imaginary play is so good that it now supersedes that of his peers. He acts out scenes from *The Lion King* or *Snow White and the Seven Dwarves* with so much passion and expression, bringing all the characters to life.

His imaginary play is over the top and he's going to be an actor for sure.

MANDING AND TACTING

Aaron was building his language bank and we were tracking the rate at which he was manding – requesting things he wanted. Manding is one of the first steps in language development and required him to communicate his needs – 'I want juice' or 'I want car'. Aaron was doing this, albeit to a limited degree. However, he wasn't tacting – commenting on his environment, as in 'Look, Mommy, there's a dog.'

A typically-developing three-year-old child will mand or tact up to 200 times an hour. We were looking to achieve 40–60 instances per hour of instructor-prompted manding as a start. We also tracked Aarons' spontaneous mands to see how fast they improved.

In order to get Aaron to learn how to comment on his environment, we hid all his favourite toys around the garden. As we walked past the bushes where we had placed them, we pointed out the hidden toys. He was delighted with the process and commented on each hidden item joyously.

The treasure hunt had taught Aaron how to tact, and he spontaneously began to point out new and interesting things in his environment.

Following instructions

Aaron's ability to understand an instruction – and to follow it – was important to his language development. In the beginning, the language concepts he was missing stopped him from being able to follow instructions.

We began by teaching Aaron simple one-step instructions such as 'Stand up!' and 'Sit down!' Once he could follow those, we moved on to two- and then three-step instructions: 'Go to your room, put on your shoes, and come to the car.'

From here, the next step was to increase the distance between the place where Aaron received the instruction and the place where he carried out the instruction: 'Go to the kitchen and ask Eli for an apple.'

These days we can give Aaron multiple instructions, which he completes with ease.

Play dates

Aaron wanted to play with other children but didn't quite know how to initiate this interaction. He'd also not yet realised how enjoyable this could be.

After a couple of play dates, Aaron started to realise how much fun he could have with other children and he paid more and more attention to what the other child was doing. Soon we no longer needed his date to entice Aaron with toys. Of course, the play skills we'd taught Aaron were also important in ensuring his social success: if he couldn't play with toys appropriately or if he didn't understand role-playing, he'd struggle to establish and maintain friendships.

As the weeks passed, we stepped back as Aaron and his play date became friends. This didn't happen overnight. We organised the play date for many weeks, setting Aaron up to be successful. Most important was for Aaron to learn from a typically-developing child. Aaron's play date was the perfect model and he began to imitate his friend. They formed a close bond.

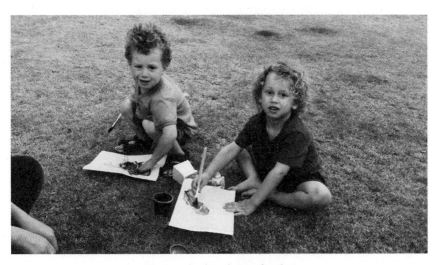

Aaron and a friend on a play date

Carolynn had advised us to get a 'bossy kid' to have play dates with Aaron. We needed a child who wouldn't give up on instructing Aaron and who'd be assertive in ensuring he sometimes played games *they* wanted to play, not just the games *he* liked.

I felt very nervous securing play dates for Aaron. The fear of rejection was always at the back of my mind and when I sent out a message asking a parent for a play date, I held my breath waiting for their reply. It made me feel very vulnerable to arrange those play dates as I'd end up comparing Aaron against his peers, which was hard. Moreover, I could barely manage to look after my own three children and felt extremely responsible about taking care of someone else's child.

My team knew I couldn't be left alone with Aaron and his play date for longer than a few minutes or I'd freak out completely. There would also be those typical demands of trying to please the play date. 'Ilana, I don't want a yellow straw – can you go get me a green one?'

'No,' I wanted to yell, but instead found myself saying 'of course' and running to the kitchen to tend to their every whim. This, however, was a small price to pay.

Today Aaron is the most social little boy ever. Nothing pleases him more than knowing friends are coming around to play – especially little girls. He even invents games for them around Cinderella characters and golden coaches – using garden chairs and string!

The next goal would be to ensure Aaron's social success in a school environment. We kept careful records on how long he engaged with his peers and extended this goal in terms of a school environment.

There were so many skills we needed to work on …

Why? and other questions

By now, Aaron was able to ask for things in order to have his basic needs met and could use language to point out items around him. With these prerequisite skills in place, it was now time to develop his language skills even further.

A big step for Aaron was feeling comfortable and confident enough to approach a classmate and ask what they were doing or where they were going. In other words, learning how to start conversations, which ultimately would lead to social interaction.

We then taught Aaron a long list of questions, breaking them down into 'the five Ws and an H' questions (what, where, who, why, when and how) to make his communication more effective. For example, he needed to be able to ask where something was located; or who it was he needed to talk to about a particular issue. Each of these simple words was a vital tool in Aaron's communication armoury.

We would systematically set up scenarios to get him to master each question word in turn. We'd hide something behind the instructor's back, saying, 'I have something/a surprise for you.' Aaron was taught to give the response 'What is it?' and was rewarded not only with the answer but with the item itself. This first step helped to pair the information and the item, to show him that the information on its own was also valuable.

We'd ask Aaron to give us the names of items he knew and of some he didn't know. The key to success here was to find a way to motivate him. This was all about matching pictures with text so he'd associate the word with the picture. Since Aaron loves animals, we did this by reading a book featuring animals he didn't know.

Aaron has always been good at reading, so we felt the animal books he loved would be an effective method to teach him. Once he'd learnt to ask a variety of questions under each category, we'd test his skills across a range of settings (in the classroom, on the playground) with a variety of people (his teachers and friends/school mates) to make sure he'd really grasped the concepts.

Children generally start to ask 'Why?' around the ages of two to three years. This form of questioning develops in complexity and understanding as they get older, and promotes a child's inquisitive nature. It leads to their understanding of how things around them are interconnected.

To avoid teaching the 'why' questions in a rote manner, it was important for Aaron to have an understanding of how things happened as they unfolded, with one thing leading to or having an effect on the next. In other words, of cause and effect. We did this by getting him to understand words such as 'before' and 'after' while involving him in the organisation of an event or activity consisting of various stages. In the beginning we got him to arrange picture cards in a sequence and later got him to tell us how the various stages unfolded. Once he'd mastered this, we looked at teaching him to answer those all-important 'why' questions before asking them. This was done through the cause-and-effect lesson, starting with simple concepts that got more complex as we went on.

At the earlier levels, we needed to ensure that Aaron had already mastered language skills such as naming objects, people and actions, and using pronouns. We started with simple concepts such as knocking over a cup and asking him why the floor was wet or dropping a block tower and asking him why the tower had broken. At first this strategy didn't work so well for Aaron as he'd focus on the effect of the action, rather than the cause (the 'why' of the activity). We shifted focus by asking him: 'What happened when I pushed the cup?', expecting him to talk about the wet floor. This did the trick – he finally got it and explained to us that the floor was wet because the cup had fallen over.

We soon realised we didn't have to teach Aaron to ask 'why' questions anymore, as he picked up the skill and made it his own, regularly requesting information about his environment.

We carried on breaking barriers one by one as we fought for him to catch up. Thousands upon thousands of hours of ABA had gotten us to this point, and we applauded this fundamental milestone in his language development.

Taking a joyous look at how far we've come

THE SWEETEST SOUND

Today, when Aaron talks, it's still a symphony concert to my ears. I crumble when he says anything. When Aaron sings, which he loves to do, my heart bursts with pride. One of his favourite songs is 'Somewhere Over the Rainbow'. His face lights up as he sings the words – to great applause, of course.

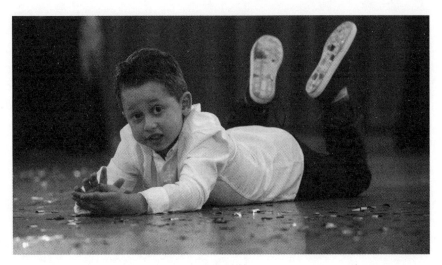

Aaron in 2017

AARON THE SHOWMAN

When Eli had his bar mitzvah, five-year-old Aaron made a speech. What a moment! He said:

> Good evening ladies and gentlemen, welcome to Eli's bar mitzvah party. I am Eli's little brother Aaron. Tonight's party is all about fireworks and with me around there's always fireworks. One day when I grow up, I'm going to have a big black belt in karate just like Eli.

Could we ever have dreamt such a day would come? Singing *and* giving speeches was beyond anything we could have imagined. These days Aaron expresses himself through the stage and has even enrolled in drama classes. He loves to go to musical shows, ice shows – any theatre, in fact.

MOM, MY FOOT HURTS

For Aaron simply to be able to tell us when and where he's sore – to express the pain he's experiencing – helps a huge amount. Every time he says 'my ear/stomach is sore', we can respond appropriately because he can identify what's wrong. With David, we never knew what the issue was; and, by and large, still don't.

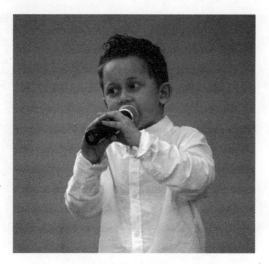

Aaron speaking at Eli's bar mitzvah

When vocal speech doesn't develop in a child, you can't fully appreciate its importance and power. This type of experience also makes you realise how intricate language is: a child can't just spontaneously have a conversation.

It wasn't only what Aaron could say that was important – successful communication depended as much on his delivery and the speed at which he spoke as on the content. Over time, our focus shifted to these equally important aspects.

Language fluency was crucial too, which meant that Aaron needed to retrieve the information fast enough and then express it fluently. Articulation, fluency and language content – all of these were key considerations.

THE SWEETEST WORDS OF ALL

Aaron was three-and-a-half when he told me for the first time that he loved me. I was putting him to bed and, a couple of seconds after he had turned over to go to sleep, he sat up, looked at me and said, 'I love you Mom.' In that moment, I knew we'd won the battle against autism. There are so many skills a child needs to have in order to be able to produce that statement. 'I love you' is quite an abstract concept. To this day, this is something David has never been able to say. It is too abstract for his understanding.

OUR INQUISITIVE AARON

Today Aaron doesn't stop asking questions and I make a point of answering each one. If I don't give him a satisfactory answer, he'll persevere and push me for more information and answers on why he can't have something or go somewhere. But every single question is like music to my ears. As Jacky arrived at school with him one morning, he watched the cars leave the school parking lot and asked her: 'Jacky where's everyone going?'

'I think they're going to work,' she answered.

His reply was precious. He said: 'Jacky, what work do you do?' Jacky had been his school facilitator for three years. Clearly, she'd done an excellent job of not giving away her role!

'Mommy, why are you crying?' he once asked me.

'Because I'm sad, Aaron,' I explained.

'Please don't cry, Mom – do you want a tissue?'

Just the other day, he asked me: 'Mom, why does David struggle to talk – he's too quiet?'

This was a particularly difficult question for me to answer. I thought about it and replied: 'Just like Moses's brother Aaron in the Bible spoke for him, you too were destined to speak for your brother David.'

Martin also has the utmost patience when answering Aaron's ever-increasing questions. 'Daddy, why is it raining?' he asks from the back of the car.

'Because the plants and animals need water to drink when they're thirsty,' Martin explains.

We've learnt that when he asks: 'Daddy, are you angry with Mommy?' when he hears our voices raised, we need to get over our argument and move on so as not to upset him. He reminds us about what really matters, and often we don't even remember why we were angry in the first place.

'Can I go to the zoo?' is a regular question, and we regularly find ourselves walking around the Johannesburg Zoo. 'Why did the sun go to sleep?' 'Will you be here in the morning when I wake up?' 'Can you sit with me? I'm scared of the dark.' These are all examples of questions Aaron's asked. Time and time again we're surprised by his questions and very often have to be creative in answering them.

Other parents may get annoyed or irritated by the number of questions their kid may be asking. But in our home each question is cherished, as we know how hard Aaron worked to achieve this all-important developmental milestone.

CHAPTER NINETEEN

DAVID'S CRIPPLING ANXIETY

'Cherish the children marching to the beat of their own music. They play the most beautiful heart songs.' – Fiona Goldsworthy

David's nervousness about change – especially any change in his daily schedule – affected how he behaved and caused him deep emotional suffering. He relied on a visual schedule to know what his day would look like, but this helped him only up to a point. Most of the time, he became so worried and fearful about what was coming next that his anxiety became debilitating, making him depressed and irrational. David would experience a sudden surge of fear, and at times like that his panic was clearly visible in his eyes. It was heartbreaking to hear him ask us repetitively what was coming next, which he did until the day ended. And he had no escape from this anxiety even then, as he would start obsessing over the schedule for the next day.

An airport experience

A particular experience of anxiety still vivid in my memory happened at the airport on our way back from our December holiday in Mauritius in 2015. We were waiting to board our flight and David's anxiety was building. Being flexible was a skill he was yet to acquire. As his anxiety rose, we desperately tried to calm him down using all the 101 ABA principles of behaviour management. Unfortunately, it was too late for those to work.

David beat himself up continually as I witnessed the gasps and disbelief of the crowd sitting around us on the airport benches. This went on for at least an hour. He was 13 years old at the time and it was quite a sight to see this type of behaviour from a boy his age. After all, by this age parents should have taught their child the proper way to behave, right?

I felt as if I'd left my body and was watching myself in a movie while I calmly ignored his behaviour as I'd been trained to do. I knew that if we moved him to the bathroom, he'd start screaming 'No, no, no!' at the top of his lungs, which was quite common for him to do in public and of course would raise even more concern from the people around us. Visions of being detained in a Mauritian prison entered my mind as I mulled over the correct course of action, weighing up the options available to us.

No doubt that day we were judged as parents who'd raised their child badly. Little did the people around us know about the hours and the money spent on trying to help our son; or about the sleepless nights we'd sat up brainstorming and planning possible ways to change the course of his autism.

Explaining a child's autistic behaviour to other adults

I've seen parents who carry cards explaining that their child has autism. The card is handed to people in public who are staring at the scene or violent outburst of the autistic child. I have heard of parents who make their children wear T-shirts that say, 'I have autism, please don't judge me.' I don't recommend these approaches to any parent. Such tactics shouldn't be necessary if our societies focused rather on helping children acquire skills; and addressed the underlying medical issues causing the meltdowns by providing the appropriate medical care.

I've heard of homes in underprivileged communities being painted purple to indicate that a child with autism lives there. The idea behind this is to let other families with an autistic child know that the house is a place they can go to for support. Support between parents or other caretakers of autistic children is undoubtedly helpful, but it should not be made a substitute for a proper societal response. We should rather educate our communities on autism, and assist families in accessing ABA and medical help.

The question of David's bar mitzvah

In Jewish tradition, when boys turn 13 years old, they have a bar mitzvah. According to Jewish law, they become accountable for their actions at this age. The meaning of the Hebrew 'bar mitzvah' is 'son of the law', and at 13 a Jewish boy is considered to have arrived at the age of religious responsibility.

Having a big celebration to mark a boy's bar mitzvah is customary and a big day in any Jewish family's calendar. Friends and family fly in from around the country and from all over the world to attend a bar mitzvah celebration. The bar mitzvah boy prepares for his big day at least 18 months in advance, learning to read a portion of the Torah, which is the law contained in the first five books of the Bible.

The bar mitzvah party is planned at least a year in advance. It involves choosing the theme and décor, a venue, a caterer, a photographer, a band and more. There's excitement around all these details and the co-ordination of outfits and invitations. Friends and family bring the bar mitzvah boy gifts, and it's a well-known joke amongst Jewish families that bar mitzvah money received as gifts lasts a lifetime!

A TIME OF LOSS AND EXCLUSION

I'll never forget the first bar mitzvah invitation we received that excluded David. It started off with: 'Dear Martin, Ilana and Eli'. David hadn't been invited at all. When I read the invitation, I was astonished that David hadn't been included. But it would be one of many we'd receive omitting David from the celebrations. I wondered what our so-called 'friends' were thinking when they left his name off – or whether they gave it any thought at all. To make matters worse, even family sometimes didn't invite David. I felt sad and disappointed. David had autism – not an incurable or contractable illness. Instead of friends and family raising us up and supporting us through their bar mitzvah year, we were left out.

There was no planning or preparation for David's 'big day', which we would have celebrated on 24 June 2015. We didn't choose special outfits and we received no congratulations. Friends and family didn't fly in from abroad to be at the bar mitzvah and we received no gifts at all. No one put together a fund for David or bought him anything, even though it was obvious that David's future earning capacity would be limited. There were no readings from the Torah and no family dinners to mark the special day. David wasn't able to take on religious responsibility, and from that perspective it would have been pointless to have a party. The last thing we wanted was anyone offering us congratulations.

One of Martin's longstanding business partners had a son who had been born on the same day as David. Their son would have his bar mitzvah on the same day David would have celebrated his. They didn't send us a party invitation but rather called to say they were thinking of us and admired us for our boundless strength and bravery. This was an act of kindness, and we appreciated their sensitivity.

THE BEST BAR MITZVAH GIFT EVER

When I told some friends that David wouldn't have a bar mitzvah, they'd stare at me in shock and disbelief, struggling to comprehend what I'd just told them. To not have a bar mitzvah was inconceivable to most. However, we had decided in advance that we were going to spend the money we would have spent on a bar mitzvah on something of more immediate value – a luxurious jungle gym.

Martin met with an architect and designed a jungle gym that we named 'The Teen Dream'. Instead of spending money on a party and on cousins we hadn't seen or spoken to in years and who didn't bother to come over or offer their support, we made sure that David acquired a jungle gym any teenager could only dream of.

The gym has a rock-climbing wall, ropes and trapeze swings, and became known as the finest jungle gym in all of Johannesburg. Eli was so excited by this space that he begged us for another one when his bar mitzvah came around.

Our son the expert climber

When David first started climbing trees around the age of ten years, we thought it was a really fun and normal thing for a child his age to do. Other ten-year-olds were climbing trees, and perhaps even making a treehouse. We encouraged him to climb when we went to the park, as he was getting too old for jungle gyms and this was challenging yet stimulating for him. In fact, David's balance and climbing skills were rather exceptional even from a young age. In no time, he would scale to the highest branches of the tree. I have always wondered how his gross-motor skills of climbing could be so advanced when his ability to speak was so impaired. Prior to witnessing his climbing skills, I had taken it for granted that a child as challenged as David was at forming words would also struggle with the kind of motor movement involved in climbing. But that was not the case!

The smile on his face when he reached the highest point on the tree was precious and we could sense his feeling of accomplishment. The higher he went, the bigger was the thrill he got. I would take many photos of him in the trees and he always enjoyed looking at them.

What started out as a typical healthy outdoor activity turned into an obsession for David. Very often we'd send him out into the garden to climb his Teen Dream jungle gym, which had been purposefully built to be as challenging as possible for any teenager. Somehow, though, it didn't provide David with all the thrills he craved. Most afternoons, we'd end up calling for him in the garden and looking everywhere for him. Finally, we'd hear leaves rustling and branches cracking. Casting our gaze upwards, we'd see David's head popping out of the very top of one of the tallest trees in the garden.

We're talking trees the height of a three-storey building! Parental panic often set in as we found it hard to believe he'd be able to get back down safely, but after making eye contact with us he'd obey our fierce command to 'Come down now!' Moreover, as skilful as David was at climbing trees, he impressed us even more with the lightning speed he displayed when disembarking from them. A few seconds, and he was back on the ground!

I'll never forget the reaction of one of the visiting CARD supervisors who had come to my house to conduct a workshop around David's ABA

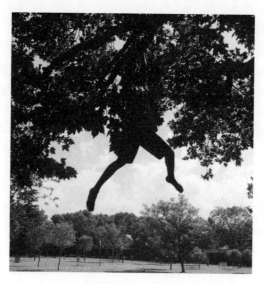

David loves climbing trees

programme. We had given David a five-minute break in the garden while we planned the next part of the workshop. Shortly afterwards, we went outside to call him in. When he didn't appear straight away I looked up and, as usual, there was his head sticking out of a treetop. The utter shock and disbelief on the supervisor's face said it all. We'd become accustomed to finding David in the trees and it was quite humorous to observe how surprised other people were on witnessing our son hanging from the highest branch possible.

We decided to enrol David in rock-climbing classes, and he has become an expert climber. Every Friday he goes to a rock-climbing barn where he climbs different obstacle courses and rock-climbing walls. He looks forward to this sport and Fridays have become the highlight of his week. I often joke that one day David will work for the army, where his strength and his talent for climbing can be put to good use scaling down and back up a helicopter rope to accomplish some mission as part of an elite unit. As long as the instructions are kept simple he will be quite capable of following through, especially since he doesn't share most other people's fear of heights.

Boat rides on the Vaal River

One Sunday, our entire family went on an outing to Zoo Lake. We hired a rowing boat and everyone excitedly jumped inside it. Martin rowed into the middle of the lake and it was precious to see how happy this outing made David feel. Aaron, too, was delighted (he enjoyed watching the ducks) and Martin came up with the idea of buying a boat. None of us believed he would actually follow through with this. Life was busy enough and boating was something that felt out of reach. Without my knowing, however, Martin started looking for a boat to buy. I'm not sure what fired him up so much – perhaps it was seeing David so happy in the boat that day at Zoo Lake – but whatever it was, Martin was determined that boating would be part of our future as a family.

After researching and investigating boats, he discovered he'd be required to take his skipper's exam and get the required licence before buying a boat. Taking the licence exam meant driving two hours to Vanderbijlpark and back to attend lessons that would qualify him. He passed his exam with flying colours, then continued to hunt for the best boat deal he could find. There was a boathouse on the Vaal River that was selling a second-hand boat and we took a drive to inspect it.

Martin wasn't entirely pleased with the boat and didn't buy it, but we'd discovered the perfect spot to store a boat once we found one. However, when Martin asked the boathouse owner if he could hire a locker for his boat, the man just laughed. He explained that lockers were impossible to come by: once someone managed to get their hands on a locker, they never let it go. A little disheartened as we had no boat and no locker, we drove home wondering whether we should forget the whole idea. A few weeks went by, and Martin decided to have another look online at Gumtree. To his surprise, he found a ski boat that was 15 years old but had hardly been used. That evening he called the owner, and by the next day had bought the boat.

When Martin arrived home the following evening, he drove through our gate with the boat attached to his tow bar. We have a fairly large driveway and were shocked when the boat barely squeezed through the gate. Martin had planned to store the boat in one of our garages but clearly this

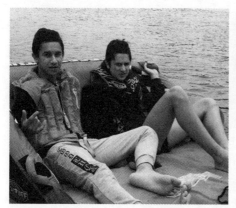 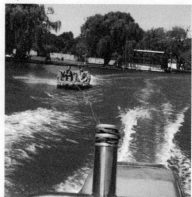

David and Eli at the Vaal River

was never going to happen. The boat was double the size of the garage! Not wanting to waste any time, Martin called the boathouse owner whom he'd met a few weeks earlier and begged him for a locker. He was not taking no for an answer! (I think he was worried about my reaction to the boat blocking our driveway.) He made a deal with the boathouse owner and we all hopped into the car late at night and made the trip to the boathouse to drop off the boat.

Every Sunday almost without fail, we pack a picnic basket, towels and swimming costumes and make our way to the river. David looks forward to Sundays and it's heart-warming to watch him sit in the front seat of the boat with the wind blowing through his hair and not a care in the world. To his delight, he and Eli get to ride on a tube at the back of the boat, bouncing over the waves at breakneck speed. It's not been easy to fill David's life with activities and things to do and the best thing we ever did for his happiness was to get the boat. On most Sundays before the boat, I'd find myself dragging him through shopping malls because I didn't know where else to take him.

Eli, too, has benefited, and will have memories of his friends joining us on the boat and of riding the waves with a happy David by his side. Almost every waking moment revolves around David and his needs, and it hasn't been easy for Eli to always have to play second fiddle to his older brother. Keeping David busy and filling his life with enjoyment and pleasure is one of the reasons we got the boat, but Sundays with family and friends at the river have also created a beneficial space for Eli – one he is able to share on a more equal footing with his brother.

In fact, going to the river every Sunday has been life-changing for all of us.

Dave's Deli

Although ABA was still the only way we could teach David new skills, he would quickly become bored, and I could sense we needed something more to fill his days. Over the years I'd learnt to become creative when coming up with new ideas for David. I thought about it and decided I'd really like David to become more independent in the kitchen. Teaching David life skills that would enhance his future ability to be as independent as possible had become a key focus and starting a deli for David popped into my mind. I mulled over it and discussed my idea with his CARD supervisor Carolynn, who assured me we could teach David how to make pizza, bake biscuits and bread, and make sandwiches to sell in his deli.

I went shopping for all the utensils David would need and designed a menu and logo for 'Dave's Deli'. The Deli has been running successfully for over a year and his team have broken down the steps to making pizza, sandwiches and biscuits into what we call 'task analysis'.

A task analysis is the process of breaking a skill down into smaller, more manageable components.

Once a task analysis is complete, it can be used to teach children or adults with autism a skill that's too challenging to teach all at once. By using prompting and reinforcement techniques, we developed a number of task analyses to teach David how to be successful in the kitchen. I had never imagined it would be possible for David to master the skill of cutting a tomato or cucumber into small cubes using a sharp kitchen knife. Tailoring David's Individual Education Plan (IEP) to target these skills has been successful, and David looks forward to his time in the kitchen.

Not only has he learnt how to bake and cook, but we also have a weekly schedule for him to follow, which helps him to check his stock and determine what he needs to buy for the Deli. On Monday mornings he'll go over his list to check on the items he needs for his menu and then go to the grocery store with one of his instructors to buy these items. This lesson has also taught David to compile a shopping list. Once David gets back from the shops, he unpacks his shopping. We've included a money lesson in his IEP so he can learn the concept of money as we're continuously working towards his independence.

David's pizza has become a favourite and so have his biscuits. We can never seem to make enough and there's never anything left over. He'll also bake bread rolls and make egg mayonnaise sandwiches that have become a popular delicacy. David can independently make pizza and the other items on his menu and will go to Martin's office building to sell his products. Each item is wrapped in brown paper with his logo – a chef holding a menu.

Since we started his Deli we've never had to contribute money to buy his stock: the money from sales has kept the concern going as David uses that to buy new ingredients.

David looks forward to making biscuits most of all and will ask me on Sundays when he's scheduled to bake biscuits during the week. He enjoys going around selling what he's made and nothing gives him more pleasure than watching people eat his food. Dave's Deli has been a great success and in the years to come we'll be teaching David new things to cook or bake that will fill his days and make him feel successful and happy. This is proof that you can create a new normal and that there's no reason why a child or adult living with autism can't lead a fulfilling life.

Sabbath and Saturday outings

David doesn't care for friends and this means once again that it's up to us to fill that void and take on the task of coming up with new ways to fill his time and keep him stimulated and engaged. He is not interested in going to synagogue as he isn't social and wouldn't really be able to participate in the prayers. Kids his age enjoy going to synagogue as it's a big social scene; or little kids like Aaron join the children's service and are kept busy with that.

Martin and I used to worry that David might create a scene at synagogue that would draw attention to him, and we got to the point where we were simply not up for it anymore.

For the family, including David, we had to create a different way of doing things on Saturdays that would work for everyone. What this would look like wasn't something we arrived at overnight – it took us years to determine what would be best for us as a family. Eli always spends the day with friends, either bringing a friend home for lunch or spending the day after synagogue at a friend's house until after Sabbath.

Sometimes I think about the fact that David has never brought a friend home or gone to spend the day at a friend's house. Other parents may not pause for even a single moment to think about this, as having friends over to play with their kids is expected. Not so for us, and so we had to design a plan for David that would be workable both for him and for us.

David's team members take turns picking him up and he goes ice-skating, or sightseeing on the Red City Bus Tour of Johannesburg. They'll also take him to play putt-putt or to rollerblade at a park. His absolute favourite place is the amusement park, as beyond anything else he enjoys the excitement and thrill of the rollercoasters. There is an outlet where he gets to bounce on different trampolines for a full hour, and Acrobranch, where he has become a skilful climber as he speeds down the zip lines and climbs the high nets and ropes around the park. David tells us in advance which outing he's chosen for the coming Saturday and looks forward to these. It's most important to us that he's happy and able to be occupied with activities he enjoys and which uplift him.

A song left unsung

For many years, thinking about when David would finally speak consumed me. In time, I got used to the silence; and then to his speaking in a different way. I never dared to dream about what his voice might sound like. I also couldn't imagine what it would be like to hear him sing. I'd often watch young kids or teens who'd entered a singing competition and it would dawn on me that David wasn't able to sing. The older he got, the more I thought about this. Something as simple as singing – a skill most children can develop effortlessly – is something David still can't do. A diagnosis of autism can be debilitating in so many ways! To have to come to terms with the fact that your child can't speak or sing, or live what you think is a normal life, is incredibly hard.

We only ever allow ourselves brief moments of sadness, however, and grab every joyful moment we can with our kids.

'Honouring David Day'

With the passing years, David's birthdays became more and more painful. Each year we'd put on a forced smile as the birthday wishes poured in. When you lose the battle against autism, all your hopes and dreams for your child's future are stripped away. On top of this, to be forced to celebrate David's birthday felt hurtful and unnatural. Taking calls and receiving messages from family members excitedly wishing us happy birthday on his behalf compounded the deep sorrow we experienced. Why wish us happy birthday? How insensitive, I'd think. 'Rather wish David,' I insistently told everyone.

David's birthday has now become a different kind of celebration. I had to find a way to ensure that David felt special on his birthday while at the same time guaranteeing we weren't forced to celebrate everything we'd lost. So, although David's birthday is on 24 June, we celebrate by *honouring* him on 22 June. Our inception of 'Honouring David Day' has been a win-win situation for everyone. He gets to be spoilt with the usual cake, presents and balloons; and we're left alone on his actual birthday, one of the hardest days in the calendar for us.

The day before his recent 16th birthday (celebrated on 22 June), I reminded David that when he woke up the next day it would be his birthday. The smile on his face when he saw his cake and balloons was heart-warming and he enjoyed every minute of us singing happy birthday and opening his presents. Tickets to the roller coaster park was the best present he could imagine and after he blew out his candles and we'd all had a slice of cake, he just sat there smiling for a while before he managed to pull himself away from the birthday table.

Instead of wishing us happy birthday, family and friends have rather wished us happy 'Honouring David Day' and sent us inspirational messages encouraging us to never give up!

David's team reflect on their journey

ASHLEIGH NIENABER, BCAT

My passion has always been to work with children who have been through a traumatic experience. When I came across The Star Academy, I realised my calling was in a different line – still working with kids, but those with different needs.

I started at The Star Academy in 2014 and the life lessons I've learnt from all the kids I work with there will stick with me forever.

David: my greatest lesson

In particular, there will always be one little boy who taught me the most. I started working with David in May 2014 and when I look back all I can remember thinking was, 'Wow, this boy really needs my help. I'm going to help him and give him everything I can.'

David had a few words but spoke mainly on his iPad, which in some cases helped him a lot but I always had this feeling it was frustrating him, as on some days he just couldn't get out what he wanted to say. There were many days I thought: 'If only I could get David to talk, how much easier his life would be, how much less frustrated he would be.'

During sessions with David I pushed him to the maximum, to the point where he'd engage in challenging behaviour such as head hitting and nose wringing because he'd had enough but didn't have the means to tell me. I'd tell him that if he was done or needed a break, all he needed to do was say 'done' – one word. This is something anyone else takes for granted, but for David it was very difficult to say just that one word.

The words are there

I started to realise that David could actually say more sounds than I thought. I'd sit with him on his beanbag during session time and say: 'David say *m*, say *b*, say *n*', etc. There were some sounds he did struggle with but the majority of the alphabet he could say. From that day I decided there's no way he can say all these sounds but can't put them into words – that didn't make sense to me at all. After that, every session we had together I'd push him to at least try one word. It didn't have to be perfect – just understandable. David trying was perfect enough for me.

At the age of 13 he was just realising his own potential and it was overwhelming for him on some days. These were the days when he just wasn't feeling 100 per cent well and giving his all was a little too much for him. On those days, I slacked off a bit but I never backed down. I told David that I understood it was difficult for him but he needed to try, that's all I wanted – for him to try. In the end he gave me his best approximation for a specific word and it was great.

A breakthrough with sounds

I made a list of sounds David struggled with and we were working on these one by one. The sound that most sticks out for me is *sh*. I started teaching David this sound in September 2015 and he said it for the first time in May 2016. At 13 years old, David learnt how to say the sound *sh* and now can use this sound in words.

I used the techniques from PROMPT to try and teach David how to say this sound. I looked at my manual and, somehow, he just wasn't learning this motor pattern properly. Until one night, feeling frustrated during a late session with David on trying to form the sound *sh*, I went to the mirror in the bathroom and looked at my own mouth. How do I say *sh*? Where is the placement of my tongue, my lips? Finally, I found a way to show David how to say this sound. David and I went back to his station, sat at the table and I said, 'Right boy, we're gonna do this now, I think I've got it.' I put my fingers next to David's lips so that they were slightly open, used my other fingers to keep his jaw closed and said: 'Say *sh*.' Right there, at that very moment, David gave his first approximation of *sh*.

I screamed out from joy and David sat in the chair with the biggest smile on his little face. This was the most beautiful moment, as he'd accomplished something we'd been working on for nine months. I jumped up and gave him the biggest hug and from there we worked on fading the prompt I'd used so he could say it independently.

David's changed behaviour

David was still engaging in a lot of self-injurious behaviour and aggression during this time, which would push him back a few steps. In 2017 David consulted with a doctor from America and I asked Ilana if I could join the consultation as I actually wanted to be part of every aspect of David's life; the more I knew the more I could try and help. This doctor cracked the biomedical side of things for David and made him feel 100 times better. His behaviours decreased; he was so much calmer; he accepted every input aimed at making him the best he could be. He was a changed boy, completely!

From then on, we were able to teach David even more than we had before because he was just taking it all in. We're now focused on his vocals and adding everything we can to get David to use his voice independently, from naming colours of items, to days of the week, to walking around the centre and naming random objects, reading books, working on sounds he still struggles with. Each week we try to teach him ten new words. This helps him learn different motor patterns. I don't think David ever thought he would be where he is today with the vocals. The smile this boy has when he gives us a word on his own or his best approximation of a new word is the most heartwarming smile ever.

David has taught me that no matter what the problem/diagnosis/ issue is, you should never ever give up on what you have faith in. Even if you don't see the potential in something, try it out, give it a go. Potential is in each and every one of our kids.

CANDICE BRITZ, BCAT

Working with David: a life-changing experience
David was one of the first children I worked and trained with at The Star Academy. I met David on my first practical training day, in 2014. He was 12 years old at the time.

I haven't seen anyone else work as hard as he did to produce whatever sound or word we were working on. David was great at communicating through his iPad, but we were focusing on getting him to use his voice more. Everyone knows how frustrating it is when you have a cold and lose your voice – now imagine this feeling reinforced tenfold. David put in 150 per cent effort in his speech but only got out a mere fraction of this. I'm surprised he didn't flip tables over and break doors, as I'm sure that would be *my* reaction. But we stuck with the programme and he really grew from this. Over time it gradually became easier for him to plan the sounds and words.

Sometimes his word production would be skewed because he was smiling so hard and you could really see the confidence in him and how happy he was with his progress.

Our BIPs for David changed frequently because his behaviour was erratic. There were often spikes in self-injurious behaviour, when Dave would hit his head using his hands and squeeze his nose so badly he left bruises. We learnt that, when there was a spike in this behaviour, that was usually a sign of something else going on with his health.

David's obsessions
David went through a phase during which he would develop a skill or a behaviour and for a time would obsess over it. The most interesting one was taking photos. There was one particular Monday morning when Ilana brought him in and said he'd taken over 1 000 pictures over the course of the weekend. I thought it was quite funny and charming – until I was tasked with the duty of deleting them. He'd run out of space on his iPad, which was his main means of communication,

and it was freezing. I remember David not being very amused with my deleting all his pictures.

I also remember observing his behaviour with pictures he'd taken: he would zoom all the way into the picture and really study it, as if he were seeing something I wasn't able to. He'd take a picture and spend minutes just studying it really closely while it was zoomed in. He'd go over every detail in the picture and didn't take kindly to being disturbed while doing this.

Working at The Star Academy was such a privilege and honour for me, and David became my best friend. He has taught me so much about patience, love and perseverance. He's truly a blessing to everyone who comes into contact with him and I'm so grateful to have been part of his life and for him to have let me into his world and allowed me to form an unbreakable bond with him. I'm so proud to see all his achievements and I can't wait to see what else he is going to achieve in his life. What a special young man he is …

CHAPTER TWENTY

MARTIN'S CANCER SCARE

Parenting children with autism is a very different kind of parenting. It demands constant emotional fitness, endurance and superhuman strength. After autism came knocking, there was very little space for any of our own physical ailments. Martin and I had to steal time for any doctor's appointment we had to make. I was hardly ever sick, which was just as well as I simply didn't have the time to pause. If I got a sore throat or even flu I brushed it off, ignoring it as if it weren't even there. The pain of a sore throat could in no way compete with the pain of my broken heart, and seemed as nothing in comparison with autism and all the experiences and worries that accompanied it. Somehow, I'd find extraordinary physical strength to carry on.

In the end, however, difficulty sleeping, becoming run down emotionally and physically, 24/7 caregiving and insurmountable challenges bringing on non-stop stress and anxiety eventually take their toll, as they did on us.

Martin wanted to make sure he'd be around to help me raise the kids and took his health very seriously. He'd never smoke or do anything to harm his body in any way. Having grown up in a home where a cold or a flu was a big deal, he'd make sure to have a yearly check-up at a physician to ensure his health was in tip-top shape. He ate well, exercised regularly and in general was fit and healthy all round.

Tinnitus and dizziness

For many years, Martin suffered from a condition called tinnitus. He would have dizzy spells during which he felt so dizzy he threw up. These were so debilitating he'd have to lie down, because if he stood up it would feel as though he were on a ship riding on stormy seas. And lying on his bed, far from being relaxing for him, was stressful in the light of the constant demands made on him.

It had all started when his ears had begun to ring continuously. The first couple of nights, we searched the room for the supposed gadget that was making the ringing noise. We looked under the bed, in the cupboard and even called an electrician to check the electrical board as the ringing sound Martin was hearing wouldn't go away and we couldn't locate its source.

After a few consultations with a number of doctors and ENT specialists, he was officially diagnosed with tinnitus. The most common cause of tinnitus is damage to and loss of the tiny hair cells in the cochlea of the inner ear. This tends to happen as people age and can also result from prolonged exposure to excessively loud noise. A frightening side effect can be loss of hearing.

Martin and I noticed that his dizzy spells seemed to coincide with particularly stressful periods in our autism battle. The reality for parents of autistic kids today is that both parents have to work to meet the financial demands this diagnosis brings. Very few families have the luxury of one person staying home just to focus on the intensive treatment plan. The world goes on while you're expected to carry out what feels like an endless and overwhelming list of priorities.

Like me, Martin juggled many things: working, supporting me and the kids and spending hours at night attending to his The Star Academy support role. Almost every day was a challenge. Medication was prescribed to alleviate the symptoms of his tinnitus, but nothing really made a significant difference.

Although truly uncomfortable, tinnitus is by no means life threatening and Martin just lived with it, fighting his way through the dizziness and nausea when the spells poked their heads into our lives.

An MRI picks up something

Martin's physician recommended an MRI to check there were no growths on the brain causing the dizzy spells, and the report came back clear. Despite the result, his spells quite soon became more intense and more frequent. This development was at the back of Martin's mind for a while and he began to be concerned that he was overdue for a follow-up MRI. Feeling nervous about the procedure's possible results, however, he put off making an appointment. The delay hung over us like a dark cloud in the weeks leading up to the second MRI.

In March 2016, the day for what we tried to think of as 'routine tests' finally arrived. The ENT had asked for an MRI and a neck scan. I'll never forget the call from Martin that left me cold and worried. 'Something is definitely wrong,' he told me over the phone. 'The radiographer was scanning my neck and then stopped and went to call the doctor. She told me she might be seeing something on the scan but wants to check with the doctor.' Although I was frozen on the other end of the phone, I told him not to worry as I was sure she was just being cautious and it was 'nothing'. I was wrong.

Fifteen minutes later, I got another distressed call from Martin. The doctor had confirmed he could see a growth on his thyroid. Surprisingly, this was completely unrelated to his tinnitus condition. Martin was told to return to the hospital the next morning so the doctor could insert a needle into the growth and collect a biopsy sample to send away for testing. The doctor explained that he needed to rule out cancer, which was a real possibility. My life flashed before me. This must be some sick joke, I thought. Cancer! How many people were there who had to wrestle with both autism *and* cancer? 'It simply can't be true!' I told myself.

Waiting in anguish for the diagnosis

I dropped what I'd been doing and sped off to the hospital to be with Martin, but by the time I got there he'd already left. I wasn't thinking straight. Worry and fear overwhelmed me as I digested the word 'cancer'. If they had found a growth on his thyroid, I wondered, had the MRI picked up any irregularities or growths on the brain? I drove home in a daze. When I arrived, Martin came out with the MRI report in his hand. Thankfully, no abnormal growths had been detected on his brain. This was something of a relief.

I tried to focus on learning more about the function of the thyroid and of course the first place I went to was Google. I typed in thyroid cancer and treatments. We had a long discussion after dinner and convinced ourselves that in all likelihood it was nothing and that the next day Martin would get a clean bill of health.

Awaiting the test results, we felt frozen in time. Even though we went about our days as normal, I had a niggling feeling that caused my stomach to turn over and over again. As the biopsy had been done on a Friday, we'd only be getting the test results back on Monday – which left the entire weekend for us to play the 'What if?' game. It was torture.

We process what we are told

Monday finally arrived and I felt sick to my core. I prayed extremely hard that we would hear good news. Martin had never missed a day of work in his life, but stayed home that day waiting for the results. Close to lunch time, the ENT finally called Martin with the news. The test had revealed that the growth was in fact cancerous. It looked like stage 1 – papillary carcinoma. We were gutted. Martin could hardly speak. The doctor asked that we come to his rooms to discuss the options. Martin was afraid he wasn't giving him all the information and we wondered why he wanted to see Martin in person.

We arrived and sat together in silence in the waiting room. When the doctor saw us, he spoke in a confident and direct manner. He began to explain the type of growth involved, and gave us his analysis of the scenario presented to him by Martin's results. He started to draw a picture, but in the middle of his diagram and explanation his phone rang. Before he picked up the call, his last words were 'but in your case the problem is … '. The seconds during which he took the call felt like hours. I couldn't breathe. Martin began to sweat and to breathe heavily. I tried to calm him down, but we now prepared for the worst.

It seemed the cancer had spread to Martin's neck. The doctor proceeded to do a scan of his neck and showed us on the screen a white mass he called a growth that would need to be surgically removed. He suspected that the tumour had spread from the thyroid to the neck. His exact words were: 'We'll need to clean out your neck.'

Martin had two options. The doctor could remove half his thyroid while taking samples from the other side of the gland during surgery. If the test results were positive, a second operation would remove the rest. Alternatively, he could remove the entire thyroid – which might be unnecessary but would mean that Martin would have to be on replacement thyroid hormones for life.

Another complication was that the muscles of the voice box were very close to the growth. The doctor cautioned us but said he'd do his very best not to 'nick' the muscle. If it *were* damaged during surgery, it would affect Martin's ability to project his voice. We requested that the operation be booked for the very next day but the first available opportunity was only three days later, with Martin last on the list of patients. We'd have to check into the hospital at 7 am and he'd only be operated on at 3 pm or 4 pm that afternoon.

An uncertain future

We were happy to go ahead and the surgery was booked. They told us that after a few weeks of post-op recuperation the next step would be further tests to determine whether the cancer had spread to any other organ. I just couldn't imagine how we'd get through waiting for these results. If it could spread to the neck, was there a chance it had spread to the lungs or – even worse – the liver? These were unanswered questions we were not going to solve, especially since we had to rush home in time to prepare for the Sabbath. I called my mother from the car and asked her to buy us tranquillisers from the pharmacy.

We arrived home and tried desperately to simply carry on with our daily routine. We tried not to give anything away, hiding our worry from the kids. That night I struggled to fall asleep and woke up in the early hours of the morning to find Martin awake too. We lay there facing the reality of what we'd just been dealt. Martin began talking about dying and his hope to be around a few more years to help me grow the kids. If only Eli had been a bit older, this would have been easier. I don't think anyone is ever ready for cancer when it knocks on the door. There's simply no 'good time' for it. Our life came to a halt and everything was immediately put on hold. We discussed the possibility of the cancer having metastasised to other parts of the body and actually managed to convince ourselves this was a strong possibility. Martin came face to face with his mortality. Trying to be brave, he spoke about all the good things in his life and what he was grateful for. I was crushed and heartbroken.

The next day was one of the hardest days of my life. I got out of bed with eyes swollen from crying and I didn't stop crying. I cried and cried for the rest of the day. The tears rolled down my face and I had no control over the deep sobs that escaped my body. We held out very little hope that things would turn out all right and it was very challenging to stay positive.

Bernie, Martin's business partner, had recently lost his wife to cancer but, once again, as he'd done years before when David was much younger, he offered a helping hand, raising us up and encouraging us to dry our tears. 'Be positive,' he insisted. 'Thyroid cancer is one of the most treatable forms of cancer.' He reminded us that we had reached our sad conclusions on our own, and that these were not necessarily based on the facts. 'Block it out and have faith,' he enjoined us.

Holding onto his words of hope, I stopped crying for the first time, dried my tears, pulled myself together and put on my brave face. By this time, Eli had gathered that Martin wasn't well and that we were both very concerned. We played it down, trying not to worry him. We told him Martin would be going in for a very routine procedure and avoided the word 'cancer' at all costs. As much as we tried to protect him from being affected by the news, however, months later Eli would show symptoms of post-traumatic stress.

Martin goes under the knife

I didn't sleep at all the night before Martin's thyroid operation, and neither did Martin. As much as I tossed and turned trying to get comfortable, I couldn't sleep. The overwhelming worry was simply too fierce to allow for sleep. Every minute felt like an eternity. The next morning, we arrived at the hospital on time and filled out the normal paperwork. Martin was shown to a bed in the prescribed ward and lay there waiting to be wheeled into theatre. I'd never seen Martin so defeated before. It was horrible to watch the distressed look on his face. We were still deciding whether to remove only part of the thyroid or the whole gland. We'd consulted our GP, who'd been in a similar situation a few months back. He'd chosen to have half his thyroid removed and the biopsy results on the other half had turned out to be benign. Martin, however, couldn't imagine going through another operation and we took the final decision to remove his entire thyroid.

We'd agreed with the doctor that Martin would be admitted to ICU after the operation. If he had a dizzy spell because of his tinnitus and needed to throw up, he would risk tearing the stitches in his neck. They put Martin on an intravenous tranquilliser in the hope he wouldn't suffer a bout of tinnitus after the operation.

In order to remove the thyroid, the surgeon makes an incision across your neck that looks as if someone took a knife and slit your throat. We were told the wound would heal and that scar cream would help. We then sat, imprisoned by time. The seconds ticked by and we waited and waited for Martin to be wheeled into theatre. Eventually, the team arrived to take him downstairs. The anaesthetist came to introduce herself and I felt confident he'd be in good hands. Saying goodbye to Martin before he was wheeled into the operating room was heart-wrenching. He gave me a reassuring nod and told me not to worry.

How could I not worry when he was about to have his neck slit open?

Support arrives with a friend

I went to sit outside the theatre. Clutching the Book of Psalms, I felt alone, helpless and worried. I tried to focus my thoughts on prayer but it was hard to concentrate. I was physically and emotionally exhausted. I prayed that the surgeon's hand would be guided and that the operation would be a success. I didn't feel confident in my prayers but did the best I could. My close friend Sandra had offered to sit with me but, being my usual strong self, I'd refused her offer. In hindsight, sitting alone waiting for the doctor to give me the news hadn't been the best idea ...

Thankfully, Sandra decided to ignore my insistence that I didn't need anyone to be with me and arrived at the hospital. She bought me something to drink and barged into the nurses' station, insisting they ask the anaesthetist to update me on Martin's status. She held my hand and soothed the pain. Sandra was there to comfort me during one of the most challenging and nail-biting times of my life. She took control and helped me through it.

Two-and-a-half hours into the operation, I had a call from a close family member asking if I needed anything. I thought they were joking and couldn't believe they'd asked me the question. I asked myself why they weren't sitting next to me outside the theatre. They'd had a birthday party to attend, which was scheduled at the same time as the operation ... Not wanting to put themselves through any kind of ordeal, they'd chosen the party. I struggled to come to terms with this but had to reconcile myself to the fact that different people handle difficult things differently. This wasn't easy to do ...

I received an SMS from the anaesthetist to let me know all was going well. I had a moment's relief and felt more positive, but of course I wouldn't be at peace until I'd had the opportunity to hear from the surgeon that he'd removed *all* the cancer; hadn't damaged Martin's voice box; and had made sure Martin was totally stable.

So far, so good

The doctor finally appeared in the hallway and I jumped out of my seat. It was good news. He'd managed to remove the thyroid without any complications. He'd 'cleaned out' Martin's neck as planned, and no other growths had been found. The growth he removed would be sent to the lab for a biopsy but Martin was in a stable condition and would soon be wheeled into ICU. I thanked the doctor and went to find Martin, breathing a huge sigh of relief after a step or two.

When I arrived at Martin's bedside, he had an oxygen mask over his mouth and was hooked up to machines that were monitoring his heart rate and blood pressure. He was awake and whispered that he'd been struggling to breathe. 'I can't breathe,' he told me anxiously. The anaesthetist arrived to check on him and told me that Martin had repeatedly complained of not being able to breathe. She'd not found any reason for his insistent claim, but had ordered a chest X-ray just in case. The X-ray would also rule out any spreading of cancer to the lungs.

After the anaesthetist had left, Martin continued to insist that he couldn't breathe. 'Come closer,' he whispered. 'Don't believe what they tell you – I can't breathe.' I didn't know who to believe or what to think. I called the nurse over to make sure, and she reassured me that he was breathing and that he'd feel better as the anaesthetic wore off. The surgeon came over to check on Martin one last time. He removed the mask from his face and asked him to say something. Martin spoke a couple of words softly and with some effort, but we could hear what he was saying. 'Great,' the doctor said calmly. 'I didn't damage his vocal cords.' He gave Martin a thumbs-up and left.

I stood at Martin's bedside for the next two-and-a-half hours, unable to tear myself away and making sure he was breathing properly. Each time he woke, he'd ask me to stay and complained about his breathing. The nurse gave him a sleeping tablet, and only when he was finally sleeping did I go home. The kids had been waiting for me to get back. When I got to the house, I walked in on David screaming, crying and hitting his head. He'd been home for most of the afternoon and needed to go on an outing to calm down. He wasn't having a good week, I realised. I put the kids in the car and drove them around for almost an hour.

The car was a safe place where I could think and where David would be happy – driving had always soothed him. On the other hand, I again felt the absence of family support very keenly in that moment. You can't do it all on your own, and right then the last thing I needed was to be driving around Johannesburg at night as a lone parent.

Before getting into bed that night, I called the ICU to check on Martin one more time. The person who answered the phone said he was fine. Eventually, I allowed myself to fall asleep.

Stress taken to a new level

I rushed back to the hospital as soon as I could the next morning, unprepared for the drama that lay ahead. Martin had had a fairly good night and was feeling a little better about his breathing. Because I could see just how devastated he was from having to battle the dread disease cancer, I tried my best to lift his spirits.

Shortly afterwards one of the ICU nurses came around and encouraged Martin to go for a walk. I learnt subsequently that no patient may walk for the first time after an operation without the physiotherapist accompanying them. Martin took a few slow steps, almost immediately complaining of feeling faint. As he lowered himself onto a chair I grabbed for him, he collapsed and passed out, falling to the ground.

I'll never forget the look in his eyes or the yellow complexion of his skin as he sucked in a last breath before hitting the floor. I didn't know what to do. I'd never felt so helpless in my life. I watched frozen in disbelief as the nurse called for assistance and other nurses ran over to help him. They placed an oxygen mask over his face, and in one minute he had regained consciousness. He sat up looking dazed and confused. The nurses carried him to his bed and checked on his vitals. I was repeatedly asking Martin if he was okay but he could barely speak. I asked his ICU nurse to call a doctor. She told me his vitals were stable and no doctor was needed. That didn't make sense to me. A patient who's just had neck surgery passes out, hitting the floor and they don't call the doctor? I insisted she call a doctor. Annoyed, she left to make the call.

She returned to tell me the doctor was satisfied that Martin's blood pressure and vitals were stable and that he wasn't coming to check on Martin. It wasn't adding up; it just didn't feel right. I made a call to my local GP and told him what had happened, asking for his advice. He gave me the confidence I needed. I beckoned the nurse over and told her to call the doctor *again* to let him know I demanded he come over to the ICU ward to check on Martin. Reluctantly, and only because of my insistence, she walked away to make the call. When she came back, she told me the doctor had asked whether I could walk over to his rooms to speak to him. I didn't argue and made my way there as fast as I could.

Nurses and doctors can make mistakes

I felt uneasy leaving Martin alone, especially after what had happened, but I had no choice. I sat in the doctor's waiting room for some time and was eventually called into his office. 'Mrs Gerschlowitz,' he barked at me. 'Who is the doctor – me or you"?

I snapped back at him fiercely: 'Your patient in ICU passes out and you don't come to check on him – what kind of a doctor are you?'

'Mrs Gerschlowitz,' he sternly replied, 'I was informed your husband felt faint and needed to sit down but that he'd recuperated and was feeling better.' 'Excuse me!' I angrily hissed at him. 'Your patient in ICU, who had neck surgery yesterday, collapsed and was unconscious lying on the ground. Is that not a reason to come and check on him?'

He paused before answering, looking surprised at my information. 'Well clearly there's been a misunderstanding,' he told me, now flustered. 'I'll come over right away to examine him.'

A few minutes after I got back to ICU, he arrived to check on Martin. He then came back to see him every hour for the next few hours. The ICU nurse assigned to Martin was removed and immediately replaced with a new nurse. It became apparent that she'd not told the doctor about walking Martin without oxygen or the physiotherapist present; and had tried to cover up the sequence of events that had led to Martin collapsing.

I sat down next to Martin unable to speak. He tried to speak to me but I couldn't bring myself to talk at all. He asked me to call his brother as he felt I was in a state and needed someone to talk to. I felt utterly and completely numb. We were so lucky Martin hadn't ruptured his stitches! The doctor explained what had happened. Martin was on medication to sedate him, and this had the effect of lowering his blood pressure. When the nurse

walked him without oxygen, his blood pressure dropped even more, causing him to pass out. Immediately placing the oxygen mask back on his face
was the reason why she'd managed to revive him so fast.

Too much to deal with

When I got home that night, David was again crying and screaming. He
was refusing to eat and was hitting himself repeatedly. Each time I arrived
home from the hospital, leaving the threat of cancer behind me, I was faced
with full-on autism.

Because David kept waking in the middle of the night, he hadn't slept
properly in ages. I heard him hit his head in the early hours of the morning. Too tired to try to solve the medical cause or even to move, I ignored
it and went back to sleep.

When I arrived at the hospital the next morning, I could see that Martin
was depressed. I sat next to his bed reciting a prayer for healing, which
brought him some comfort. Physically, he was getting better, and the doctor had already moved him to the general ward. There were a few other
patients in the ward, and it struck me that they were all much older than
Martin. 'How can this be happening?' I asked myself. 'We were meant to
grow old together, so why are we going through this now?' It was difficult
to remain hopeful in the face of these feelings.

Our prayers are answered

It was a Friday morning and the surgeon had come to do his ward rounds.
He was happy with Martin and signed his discharge forms. The nurse
wheeled Martin to my car and we drove home. We'd been home a few hours
when I heard Martin gasp and call me over. I ran to check on him, expecting the worst. The surgeon had sent him a text message. He'd received the
biopsy report from the lab. The tumour on Martin's thyroid was benign.

I laughed out loud, trying to process the news. I was over the moon that
it hadn't been cancerous – meaning it hadn't spread to any vital organs.
Martin, on the other hand, had mixed emotions because he'd opted to have

his entire thyroid removed. The surgeon later explained that the nodule in Martin's neck he'd thought was cancerous was in fact an enlarged parathyroid gland. A thyroid has four parathyroids that are responsible for calcium regulation. Martin had three parathyroids left and, with the right medication, would lead a completely normal life.

When we told friends and family the news, their first reaction was to blame the surgeon for making the wrong call in removing Martin's thyroid. Yet as far as we were concerned, we had no one to blame – we only had G-d to thank for granting us a new lease on life.

Every day since the beginning of Martin's cancer scare, he and I recited a special mystical prayer. This beautiful and moving prayer is an outpouring of gratitude to G-d, and depicts our utter dependency on G-d's mercy. Not a week goes by when we don't recite the prayer in remembrance of this miracle.

This experience taught me that life is fragile, precious and unpredictable. It's on rough days like these that we have to maintain hope for a brighter morning – even through the darkest nights. Through prayer, we can change destiny.

As for the tinnitus, well … that's still there. But it's feeling a great deal more bearable for Martin than used to be the case!

CHAPTER TWENTY-ONE

AARON AND THE BATTLE FOR INTEGRATED SCHOOLING

From nursery school to Grade R: 2014–2018

Aaron's prerequisite skills for school were in place one year after we started his ABA programme and it was time to find him a suitable school placement. I strongly suspected that his inclusion in a mainstream school was going to be a challenge to secure. After all, I'd had past experience of approaching schools when I was searching for David's placement. As fate had it, I found myself once again in the position where I had to fight for educational rights.

The lawyer in me took over and I found myself buried in legislation on inclusive education. I wanted to make sure I knew my legal rights and briefed counsel to give me an opinion on the law. The conclusion was that inclusive education was a right and not a privilege in South Africa. According to the Constitution of South Africa, the South African Schools Act of 1996 and *White Paper 6, Special Needs Education: Building an Inclusive Education and Training System*, Aaron had the right to be enrolled in a mainstream school.

As much as inclusion was a legal right, however, it wasn't widely practised in schools around South Africa and much work was still needed to entrench the law.

The benefits of difference

Inclusive education values the unique contribution each student can make to the class. The opportunity for students with a difference to learn alongside their typically-developing peers in general-education classrooms has become more urgent than ever before, especially considering the increase in the incidence of the autism diagnosis.

I had all my arguments in support of Aaron being included in a mainstream nursery school carefully planned and went over these reasons a few times. Without a real understanding of human differences, how could children become complete adults capable of contributing to a healthy, fair, non-judgemental society? A society that, at its core, has a strong sense of good morals and values, *has* to encourage exposure to children with a difference. Religious schools especially, which claim to teach children good morals and values, have to be true to their mission statements.

Our South African education system tends to box children in different 'classes' with specific labels, such as 'remedial', 'special-needs' or 'school-ready'. A future where segregation along such lines is no longer a common practice was, surely, something to be encouraged and welcomed.

The time had come for me to take a stand. I was prepared to do everything necessary to change the old-school norms that placed children with a difference in their own boxes and sent them packing to special-needs schools. Reform had to be possible. Aaron deserved the opportunity to bridge his challenges. He would continue with his one-on-one programme, but also needed a mainstream school setting where he could model his peers. If the class teacher were open to it and willing to give him the support he needed, there would be no limits to what he could achieve. I was adamant that we needed to have a shift in thinking. This would entail abandoning the approach that simply identified learners who couldn't keep up with the class and shipped them off to various therapists, or to a remedial or special-needs school; and embracing a new mindset of 'Look at how I, the teacher of a mainstream class, am going to address the individual needs of each learner with a difference.' Aaron's presence in the classroom would pave the way for many other children needing a foot up in future.

An anticipated rejection

It was 2014 and time to secure a place for Aaron at nursery school. But there was a big hurdle to overcome first: meeting the principal of the nursery school we'd chosen. As I walked into her office for the appointment I'd made with her, I felt uneasy. I was going to ask her if Aaron could be included in their school accompanied by a facilitator, and I was fully anticipating her refusal.

I took a seat, feeling anxious because there was so much at stake. Even though I'd come prepared, in that moment I got stage fright and had no idea how I'd find the right words to secure my child's future. I'd rehearsed the reasons why Aaron should be allowed to attend the school, and why his presence would actually be beneficial for the school, over and over in my mind. Once I sat in front of her, however, I forgot my carefully rehearsed lines and began to be overwhelmed by fear of rejection. What if she said no? In that moment, I couldn't even remember the legislation I'd so carefully researched.

Thankfully, she was open to the idea of inclusion. When she said yes, I almost leapt out of my chair from excitement. I breathed a sigh of relief, grateful to her for supporting the idea. It was very important for Aaron's development and programme that we find a suitable school environment that would make it possible for him to learn the skills he was lacking.

Towards independence

Not only did we require a typical school setting for Aaron, but we also needed a school that would be flexible enough to allow him to go in and out of the classroom as well as spend one-on-one time with his facilitator. Carolynn explained that in general, if a child needed *more than 25 per cent* support in the classroom, a facilitator would be required. The school we had sent Aaron to was able to understand and accommodate this need.

Slowly, we built up the time Aaron spent at school. We started with him going for an hour daily, increasing the time as he gained more skills and his learning gaps closed. One of the purposes of school for Aaron would be to teach him how to transfer the skills we taught him in his one-on-one programme to a classroom environment. In order to ensure his independence at school, Aaron would also have to master a long list of goals. Carolynn had insisted that a structured class with rules would ultimately result in Aaron's independence and success.

Following instructions, staying on task, taking part in class discussions or retelling stories when asked to do so, are complex skills. Being expected to answer questions or follow instructions one on one is very different from doing those things as part of a normal classroom scenario. In a classroom, where there's so much going on with lots of distractions, the chances were much greater that Aaron might lose focus and concentration.

Our facilitators were briefed on Aaron's specific needs and worked on his daily goals. They needed to know when to step in and support him and when to step back. Finding the right balance was tricky. Ultimately, Aaron needed to learn from his peers and his teacher. As soon as he could manage on his own, learning from his natural environment, we'd do away with facilitation completely.

Blending in well

The school team worked closely with us and every week we briefed the teacher on Aaron's goals. Working in a team was important to reach Aaron's long-term goal, which was to be successful in a mainstream school without any additional support. Communication was the thread that held it all together. The teacher was responsible for a class of 20 kids, with 19 children to manage apart from Aaron. We had to make Aaron's integration process as seamless as possible, ensuring that our presence in the classroom did not make her feel uncomfortable and without imposing in any way. Our facilitator would have to win her over.

Teachers are not all open to working with a facilitator, as this means there's another person in the classroom all the time. It was also important for Aaron's facilitators to make friends with the other kids in the classroom, creating opportunities for Aaron to be included socially. If the facilitator was doing her job properly, the children would feel she was there to support the class and not just Aaron.

Jacky was excellent at school facilitation and won Aaron's classmates over in no time. If Aaron missed a day, the other children would ask where he was. We arranged many play dates so Aaron could make friends outside the classroom, making it much easier for him to interact during school.

Over the years, we worked on many school goals to secure Aaron's independence. When he was two years old, we focused on getting him to imitate his peers. We'd gather data to record the instances when he'd imitated them. When he turned three, his goals changed and we expected him to interact with his peers for a certain length of time. Working on play skills during our one-on-one sessions was key to ensuring his social success. If he wasn't able to play 'cooking' or 'hospital' or to ride an imaginary train in the classroom, he wouldn't be able to learn from his peers or maintain long-term friendships.

This intervention, made during the early foundation years, was key in shaping him for mainstream schooling then and in the years to come.

Going for gold

As time went by Aaron continued to make steady progress, but this was still always against the clock. We heeded Carolynn's warning that Aaron needed to achieve more than a typically-developing child in a year. Yet he *was* running at the right pace, with me right by his side every single step of the way. We never threw in the towel when we encountered a roadblock – even though there were many of those.

As Aaron got closer and closer to full recovery, I had to muster every ounce of my strength to make it to the finish line. Every step was agonising. At the start of a race, you're fresh and energetic, but as the miles go by you become worn down. Your muscles start to ache and cramp. The beginning of the race can be intimidating because you know what lies ahead, but the closer you get to the end the more you need to draw on your inner reserves as you've been on the road running for a long time.

From the very beginning, I was running Aaron's race to win it. I'd tell Martin that I was going for gold. Martin would respond that what Aaron had already achieved was good enough. We had gotten our boy back, and what remained to fix amounted to mere polishing and the final touches. As far as he was concerned, we'd already won gold. Although I savoured every minute of Aaron's development, however, I knew I still had to cross the finish line.

As much as the responsibilities and rewards of raising Aaron were unparalleled, being tied down to an ABA programme and a school facilitator took its toll on me. We were never free. My child was under evaluation for four years of his life. Looking back, it was worth it, especially if one considers the outcome. But it was hard. Determined, I pushed forward, surviving the hard days and the endless criticism.

In a way, I lost the freedom of his childhood and the way I'd hoped it would be. Aaron, on the other hand, enjoyed playing with his instructors. Although there were times when he had to work really hard, he had never known a different existence and so accepted his life as it was.

Still, our weekly ABA schedule imprisoned us and I longed for it to come to an end. It would be enough having to deal with David's endless issues and demands.

Insights from other members of Aaron's army

Aaron had an ideal team. Here they tell their stories and share their insights.

BIANCA CASSINGENA, BCAT

When I first laid eyes on Aaron Gerschlowitz, I knew in my heart this little boy was a miracle. I started working with Aaron ('Azi Bops') when he was only 18 months old. When Ilana asked me to be a part of their team, my heart filled with determination. This little boy was crying on the inside to fight for a chance to engage with all the opportunities life has to offer. And with two of the most driven, determined, loving and hard-working parents, this miracle was achieved.

I became Aaron's team leader a few months after I began working with him. This incredible little boy had many gifts and talents visible right from the start. I knew we were fighting; I knew we were at war and that time was against us. I understood what we were working towards and where the concerns lay.

Aaron is the gentlest and most loving soul. Kind and caring with the sweetest little smile. He wanted to please; he wanted to fight and escape the grip of autism. And boy, did he do just that.

Saving Aaron

The hours were long and the work intense but Aaron didn't give up. Neither did Ilana or Martin. Ilana and I became two soldiers fighting side by side for Aaron. We spent many hours discussing Aaron's programme, finding ways to achieve the goals set out for him and deciphering how to teach him certain programmes. His team was amazing. From his supervisors to his therapists, they all gave a piece of themselves to save Aaron.

Ilana and I spent a lot of time together. Aaron became my focus at The Star Academy and became my life. I couldn't eat, sleep or talk without thinking of him. As for Ilana, I've never met such a driven, determined and hard-working person. Her heart was broken when she first saw signs of Aaron's autism. Her worst fears were in front of her, but she didn't give in to them. She didn't surrender – the autism simply fuelled her fire, motivating her to fight these fears. Despite the knocks she experienced, including those from people who didn't believe Aaron could defeat autism, she persevered.

Having David, her eldest son, living with autism, she refused to lose her baby boy also. I remember seeing the desperation in her eyes coupled with her deep motivation and I knew I had to give my all to help Aaron. There was no other way. I decided there and then that Aaron would become my focus, not only at work but in everything.

If I had to describe the qualities that helped Aaron defeat autism, I'd say it was his positive and light-hearted nature, his resolve and his beautiful soul. To describe the journey he went through, I must start at the beginning.

Aaron's first clinic

I'll never forget when we were introduced to this beautiful little boy. I took one look at him and thought, 'Wow, it feels like I've known him before.' This was something I felt throughout my time working with Aaron. I felt our souls had already met. I understood him, not through words or behaviour but on a soul level. I'd often look into his eyes and know what he was feeling and felt he knew the same with me. During our first clinic we were given our initial tasks and programmes. The work began.

I remember my first session with Aaron as though it was yesterday. He loved small things such as beans or sand. We were attempting to work with him in a very natural way, integrating lessons with play. He took the box of beans and threw them on the floor. They went everywhere. He began playing with them, moving them around, pushing them up and down, making them move. When I tried to move him away from the beans, he'd cry his little heart out. I tried packing them away, but this would upset him even more. Sitting still was difficult for him. Eye contact wasn't completely non-existent, but according to the standard milestones he should have had more.

Transitioning (changing activities or going from one environment to the next) at times wasn't easy for Aaron. After a few sessions Ilana picked up that some structure was needed and she was right. We began moving to more structured sessions, where we'd teach Aaron at a table and reinforce his learning with some of his favourite activities. This was easy because he *loved* movies! He'd laugh, smile and giggle, pointing at the screen. You could see from this that Aaron knew exactly what was happening; that he wanted to engage and express himself ... he was trapped but wasn't giving up!

The doors start opening

We started to teach Aaron object labels, beginning with the simplest matching instruction, moving on to a receptive instruction (e.g. 'Identify an object and give it to the instructor'). Usually these steps take time for children to master, but Aaron flew through them. If he got stuck, Ilana would have us replace the objects as she realised he got bored quickly. As so often before, she was again spot on. Aaron was a fast learner, but if he got something wrong he'd get bored with the task. We'd then have to change the way we were teaching him or change the object and come back to it.

Aaron taught me flexibility and forced me to be creative when teaching him. He didn't fit into the typical ABA programme – he needed a lot of flexibility. This was a lesson for many of us in our thinking and programming. There were programmes we got stuck on, such as *o* in verbal imitation or 'arms out' in actions. Aaron, Ilana, his team and I wouldn't give up. We persevered, and he broke through.

Becoming social

We began taking Aaron to school for facilitation. In the beginning, we could see the challenges that lay ahead. Aaron didn't enjoy sitting for long periods of time. He enjoyed playing with toys but his actions were often repetitive and he preferred to sit on his own. This wasn't so much a choice: it was more about not knowing how to play with others. This was clear from day one.

Aaron wanted to socially engage; he wanted to play with toys in multiple ways and sit for a longer time to take in his environment. All we needed to do was teach him. I remember how he used to look at his classmates and smile and laugh ... If only he'd had the words to engage, if only he'd had the vocabulary to do so. My heart sank when I saw this and I could only imagine what Ilana and Martin felt when what I was feeling broke my heart. I couldn't imagine what it was like for them. This strengthened my desire to help Aaron even more.

During many hours and on many nights Ilana and I would sit reshuffling his programme, trying to figure out how best to teach him. There were some days that were harder than others for Ilana; I could see the hurt in her eyes and tried to provide comfort where I could. This although I knew no words would provide solace. Yet not once, throughout this journey, did she give up on her son ... her strength was inspiring!

No let up

I remember going away with Ilana, Martin, David, Eli and Aaron to Sun City and Cape Town. On both holidays we kept up Aaron's sessions. Recovery had no holidays or rest. The Gerschlowitzes became more than employees, more than work – they became like family.

And then suddenly Aaron began to soar and soar and soar – through each programme and each lesson. He opened up and began learning, absorbing and growing from strength to strength. This period, however, wasn't short of challenges. Occasionally we'd hit a wall and progress would be slow. I knew all he needed was time, patience and faith. When working session after session, from the perspective of a child, parents or a facilitator, these qualities can be severely tested. Looking for the positives can be very challenging, but when there are breakthroughs, whether big or small, they all feel like a significant achievement.

The pay-off

Aaron began to sit for lengthy periods and to eat foods of differing textures. He made beautiful eye contact; his motor tasks were incredible; and he began vocalising and speaking! My heart swelled with joy as he mastered one skill after another – what a champ! Tasks we'd worked on for quite some time, he suddenly conquered. Working with him was the most rewarding job: he gave, and gave, and gave. He wanted to please, to achieve – and he wanted to beat autism.

The hardest goodbye

Then the day came when I had to say goodbye to Aaron, his team, Ilana and the little family I'd formed. I was going to do my Master's in psychology and my journey with Aaron had come to an end. It was one of the most difficult decisions I've had to make in my life. I felt as though I were leaving behind a piece of myself, as though I were saying goodbye to family. Ilana and I had become so close, more than boss and employee – friends. I was devastated. I felt as though I were letting her, Aaron and his team down. I knew they would be more than okay without me as he had a wonderful team and incredible parents, but I still felt guilty leaving. I'll never forget the day I first told Ilana – we were both in tears. Not a day passed when I didn't think of Aaron or Ilana. It was so hard to stay in contact for a while, because I didn't know how to do that without giving it my all. I didn't know how to continue the relationship from a distance.

A dream come true

I went to visit Ilana and Aaron recently … I was absolutely blown away by the unbelievable progress he'd made. Full conversations, perfect social interaction – I had to ask Ilana why he was still having sessions, because to me he'd recovered. Aaron had escaped the claws of autism and he was free. My heart was beyond happy. I was elated.

Ilana was so proud of her son. I was so proud of him too, as well as of his incredible team and amazing parents. They have been with him every step of the way and the result is extraordinary. Aaron can defeat anything that comes his way. He's overcome the most difficult challenges. A little angel sent from heaven.

My angel

To the little man who stole my heart: you are the bravest person I know. You have overcome more obstacles than many people will ever face in a lifetime. You are pure light, pure joy and pure happiness. Your golden heart is a true treasure. Thank you for teaching me perseverance, faith, kindness and unconditional love, as well as how to feel without words.

To Ilana and Martin: your dedication and strength are beyond admirable. I'm so grateful Aaron has you as his parents. I have learnt true determination and strength from you both.

To David and Eli: thank you for being such incredible brothers to Aaron.

To everyone who has worked with Aaron: your talent, skills and love for what you do has contributed to this amazing miracle, thank you!

JACKY VICENTE, BCAT

I'd just finished writing a three-hour mid-year exam for my psychology degree at UJ (the University of Johannesburg), and as I walked out of the exam room, there was Ilana, who said, 'Excuse me, excuse me – please take this paper'. I took the paper, scrunched it up and shoved it in my bag because all I wanted right then was my winter holiday.

The holiday came and went, and in August we began the final stretch for the year. I cleaned out my bag and there, at the bottom, I found The Star Academy sheet. I thought: 'I don't have any money and I'm living off my mom and dad. I actually need a job!' I emailed Ilana to ask whether the job was still available.

Just a job to boost my Master's application – or not …
This was the first real job of my life, closely aligned to psychology and to working with children. I thought, 'Honours here we come … Master's here we come … and I'll be earning money!' I'd always wanted to work with children with special needs and possibly to open up some kind of care centre myself one day.

When I went to the interview in 2010, I immediately loved The Star Academy. It had just started in earnest and there were children everywhere. I did the training and wrote the exams through CARD in the United States, which was an amazing experience. I started working as a junior instructor and grew from there to senior instructor. Then my circumstances changed and I left for Portugal for nine months. When I returned, I was thrilled to get my job back and to become Board Certified.

The children steal my heart
It's the children who make me love my job; the fact that I feel a certain obligation to them although no one made me feel obligated. I feel I've been put here to give them a fair chance. It's the success with the children that's so rewarding – not the money. It's getting a child to talk, or playing a part in their learning to ride a bike or just swallow a tablet. That's pure satisfaction in itself.

Groundbreaking moments

There have been so many special moments but out of all the children I've worked with, I feel Aaron in particular is my special baby. I've known him since he was tiny and since he had his shutdown, and have proudly watched his progress. Now that he goes to school and doesn't need us I feel a little bit heartsore.

He was 17 months when I first started working with him. Two months before this, when I was planning the year-end function and talking to Ilana, she had Aaron in her arms and he was pointing and acknowledging stuff around him. She said she was so happy to see this because of her experience with David. I remember thinking, what a cute baby. I'd only been back from Portugal five months, so didn't know him that well.

The following February was when everything changed with Aaron. That's what I call 'the shutdown'. And we needed to bring him back. On the first of February Ilana called me and explained what was happening with Aaron. I felt huge empathy, as she was going through this for a second time, which was unthinkable. She said: 'Jacky, I need your help.'

Total commitment

Ilana calls me feisty – but she had faith in me from the beginning, which in turn gave me faith in her and [the ABA] process. We started working with Aaron at her house. I remember one day in particular, when I saw her cry while changing his nappy. I'd always thought of Ilana as such a strong woman, someone who would only cry behind closed doors. And there she was crying in front of me, and I thought: 'Jacky – you have to do something. You have to make this boy well again.' At the same time, I was thinking: 'I'm just one person and it's not my decision. Although it's a life-giving opportunity, maybe I'll lose my job if I can't fix my boss's child.' Then again: 'But if I *can* do it, just imagine this child's life.'

After that, Aaron and I had an instant connection. I found I could speak to him through his eyes. There was no one else he'd respond to in the same way and I'd always treat him with a very loving firmness. I would have taken a bullet for him, and he knew it wasn't him but his brain I spoke to when I said: 'Now it's time to start working.' For the first six to eight months we did the same thing every day with the same result – zero. I'd see the hope in Ilana's eyes slowly fading and felt my hope fading also. I felt the tenuous chain we had was breaking, becoming fragile. Then suddenly one day Aaron decided, 'Hello world, I'm back!' It was amazing.

The door opens
We had to get his brain to copy what we were showing him. Once he could do that he would conquer the world, because then I would be able to teach him anything. Then one day during his lesson, when I said: 'Say *br*', he started to cry. By now he hated me doing this, constantly pushing him to do something he couldn't physically do. I wouldn't stop, though. I wouldn't give up. The team just carried on doing the same thing each day.

Finally, I said: 'Okay, we're going to do talking today and I'm not going to take no for an answer.' I was completely firm in a loving way. He looked back at me in a loving baby way, while chewing on a piece of meat. And I said: 'Say *gr*'. 'Here we go again,' I thought, when I suddenly heard a raspy *gr* from his throat. I thought perhaps he was choking on the meat so I checked his throat. I swiped his mouth – no meat in there. I said: 'What's going on, are you sick?' He stared back at me as he couldn't answer. I'd always talk to him as though he was my best friend. He gave me a slight smile and I said: 'Try again – say *gr*'. And again he did his throaty *gr* and I clicked – he was trying. My whole world spun. I was overwhelmed with happiness, and fear that he wouldn't repeat it. Was I doing the right thing at this point? Would more come? Well, it did. He suddenly started talking and the floodgates opened. I even put it on video. Then he started hitting the milestones.

ABA does work

This really made me believe wholly in ABA. I told everyone: 'Look at what this can do.' Working with Aaron gave me faith for every other case. He was my project – my baby. When you work with a child for three to four full days a week, they become your family and now five years down the line I'm exactly like a proud mom.

Aaron at school

I sat with him in his first few days at school – just in case he needed me on a social level. If I was outside the class and heard a child screaming, I'd wonder whether that was him screaming again. But no, it was another child. Here he was at school – a boy who hadn't been able to talk!

We'd used PROMPT on him so his muscles could heal. He so wanted to succeed. The block on his mouth was stopping him but his brain wanted to succeed – the words wanted to come out. He tried at every opportunity. He loved movies and would do anything to get one, so we used that to our advantage in helping him to start talking. We'd pause the movie and say: 'Tell us one thing you see' and then we'd point to something and he would say 'bird' (or this or that).

A different child

Now he doesn't shut up. In the car it's 'Why this?' and 'How come that?' One day he told me: 'You need to be happy today Jacky.'

Success is all about early intervention. I've now experienced the difference. There's an optimum time for intervention. You do see progress in older children, but with Aaron it took a year to see major progress and another two years to completely catch him up.

Every case is different, and every brain works differently. It's as simple as that. Aaron wanted us to help him get out of there and, step by step, he emerged from his own world.

IANA TCHOUKANSKA, BCAT AND MASTER'S IN EDUCATION

When I first got the call from Ilana to join Aaron's team, I was over-whelmed. I'd had plenty of experience with small children but not one quite as young as Aaron (who had just turned 27 months). Ilana spoke with great enthusiasm and energy, and the one sentence I'll never forget was: 'With Aaron, we're pushing for recovery.'

At that point in my career I knew recovery was possible. This was based on everything I'd read on research into autism in the United States; and on my experiences of ABA at The Star Academy. I knew it worked. However, I hadn't seen recovery first-hand. Not yet.

When I first met Aaron, he was tiny. Although he made a num-ber of sounds and giggled throughout the first session, he was quiet overall. His vocal skill set was limited to imitating approximately 20 sounds. He had five functional words: 'bottie' (his bottle), 'mama', 'up', 'moo-ee' (for movie) and 'op' (for open). These he used to communi-cate his needs when prompted. Aaron was learning to imitate, which is important for language. He wanted to communicate. He just didn't know how.

Right from the start there was a sense of urgency. Everyone recog-nised there wasn't one second to lose. We had a purpose, a goal. If a single lesson was stagnant, we needed to figure out why. Did we have the right reinforcer – was he motivated? Was the way we were teach-ing effective? He had a big task ahead of him. Not only did he need to catch up on the skills he lacked – he also needed to learn at the same pace as everyone else.

Lessons were changed, added and removed on a weekly basis. Everyone working on the team needed to be incredibly involved. What was fantastic for me was the level of involvement from Ilana and Martin. His team did not just consist of the instructors working with him during his designated ABA hours. Aaron's teacher at school needed to be just as consistent with him. Ilana and Martin would continue with the interventions after hours. Even Eli was recruited as the official 'demonstrator' for a variety of lessons. Every area of Aaron's life needed to be consistent. He needed to know that the same expectations were placed on him everywhere. When he learnt to say 'open' rather than just relying on the syllable 'op', everyone knew, celebrated and expected that he would now use the word instead.

In the beginning phase of Aaron's programme, we pushed for articulation and imitation. I remember the day when all the team's hard work kicked in and suddenly his vocabulary was the same as that of any other child his age. I hadn't thought the day would come when Aaron's speech apraxia would stop being an issue. Now it seemed the sky was the limit.

The early years were filled with pressure and felt 'dangerous', in the sense that every step was critical. This didn't mean that the later years were any less important, only that my mindset shifted from 'if' he was going to recover to 'when'.

Aaron's lesson priorities shifted quickly. Once his echoics were strong, we worked on filling up his language content. Once he had a strong enough 'library' of language, we had to teach him the everyday use of the words. Of course, it was inevitable that there should be bumps and hurdles along the way. But knowing how we'd helped him through the toughest of times, I knew he could overcome them.

In considering the amazing journey this little boy has made, it's really important to stop and remember that it didn't all come at once. It comprised of small victories, which when put together resulted in something truly remarkable. While in isolation these accomplishments may seem minor, together they've given him the skills he needs to be successful in mainstream school. He shows us that what seems impossible is not necessarily so. ABA works: I know because I've seen it work. But it takes time and hard work. It requires commitment from everyone involved. It calls for a 'never-say-die' attitude and a willingness to turn over every stone until a solution is found.

Aaron's continued progress is testament to this. I remember how, after his first school concert, I said to Ilana that I couldn't wait to see how much further he would come by the following year. This statement continues to stand true as each year passes.

KIRSTEN WATT, BCAT

I first started working with Aaron in June 2014. He'd just turned two years old the previous month. He was the smallest person I'd ever worked with. I remember him for his gorgeous curly blonde hair and his brightly coloured leggings and tops. Aaron absolutely loved his movies. *Mickey Mouse Clubhouse, Little Einsteins, Noddy, Snow Buddies* and *Rio*. They were all his favourites and he'd sit and watch them happily for ages.

When I came onto 'Team Aaron', we were working on imitating the sound *m*. This lesson was frustrating for him. It was as if there were a missing link somewhere and he couldn't understand what he was supposed to do. I would start my session sitting on the floor in front of the mini DVD-player. Aaron's shirt was often drenched in saliva. This was because he had a hard time lifting his jaw to keep his lips together. We did exercises every 15 minutes to try to strengthen the connection between the sounds we were making and the muscles he needed in order to make the sounds. Aaron worked tirelessly on learning sounds. We focused most of his lessons on echoing different sounds, then blending these together.

Aaron spent up to six hours a day learning to speak with his instructors. We used Aaron's love for movies to help him imitate one sound at a time. At first he just imitated the sound once, but he soon learnt that saying the sound *m* meant he could watch his movie again. I'd never been prouder. He was so small and he'd worked so hard just to be able to make this single sound. Aaron kept on working hard and learnt more sounds one at a time.

Aaron the movie star
Functional pretend play was another lesson we worked on with Aaron. We'd recorded a video of team members playing with a wooden pretend pizza. We'd play a small section of the video and pause it so we could help Aaron imitate the actions he'd seen in the video. This was a really tough activity for him when we started out. He didn't seem interested in playing with the pizza, his toy animals or his cars. He

needed prompts for every single action and didn't make a single sound. Despite this, we carried on teaching him.

One day, something clicked. All of a sudden, he showed interest in the videos. He laughed at his team members making silly sounds with his cars and doing ridiculously over-the-top scenes with his Mickey Mouse toy. Now that he was interested in the videos, we were able to prompt Aaron to imitate the actions in a way that made sense to him. Soon he was imitating a whole video, then moving on to learn others. He learnt the sequences word for word and action for action. He would even request his favourites. I was amazed at how far he'd come.

Breakthrough after breakthrough
Our work wasn't done, though. We continued to teach Aaron new scenes to play with different toys. Our aim was to have Aaron become more spontaneous in both his play and language. Imaginative play became one of his strengths. He started to show a real interest in his animal toys, his cars and Thomas the Train! All of a sudden, we could use the toys to teach Aaron new words and new skills. All the frustration he'd been experiencing a few months earlier had turned into motivation and joy. Aaron had learnt how to play and I was never more excited than at that point in his development.

Soon we were using his toys to teach Aaron how to request things using full sentences. Ilana told us that we needed Aaron to start using a wider variety and larger number of words when he requested a toy or something else he wanted. I remember having to hold up my fingers each time Aaron asked for a different toy, to remind him to use three words instead of only one. This was challenging but we weren't giving up.

I was amazed, and sometimes couldn't believe that the same little boy who had struggled to say *m* for movie was now learning to ask for his toy piggy using a full sentence. Aaron's new-found love for his toys was a big motivator. His team was committed to expanding his language. By far the most committed member of the team was Ilana. She was always there to recognise when the team needed a little inspiration. She was always willing to give us whatever we needed in order to give Aaron the best chance to succeed.

I've worked with Aaron for just over three years now. Each year Aaron has surprised me and overcome challenge after challenge. As the year 2017 drew to a close, I started my session with Aaron sitting on the floor in the same spot where we'd struggled to learn the sound *m*. Except that now Aaron told me all about his day at school; what his friends had done during the day; and his favourite new toy. He also reminded me that lions are mammals and live in the Pride Lands of Africa. He spoke so much I had to interrupt him so we could start our lessons.

Aaron has worked so hard to get to where he is now. He's a passionate little boy with an infectious laugh. I've never been more convinced that he will achieve anything he sets his mind to.

Those easy labels

I was struggling to envisage the end of the ABA road, and I now began to feel as if we were fixated on grooming and creating the *perfect child*, flawless in every way. In a sense, I was beginning to have feelings similar to Martin's and I started to wrestle with my sense that we should look at things anew. It felt as if Aaron couldn't just be a child having a bad day or needing to learn new concepts and skills. The hardest part was to shake off the stigma that followed him around, the 'shadow' attached to him that moved with him wherever he went.

In the end, it proved to be extremely difficult for the school to set their expectations for Aaron. He'd started with a facilitator, which obviously indicated he'd had learning deficits. Granted. But there seemed to be little sense of his progress, or of his 'ordinariness'. The things Aaron did were not easily viewed as something any typical little kid might do. Rather, they were an indication that he had 'a problem'.

If Aaron complained about being asked to pack away the toys to start circle time, it was considered an issue, an indication that he had 'difficulty transitioning between tasks', instead of being perceived as just another instance of a five-year-old protesting about packing away toys he'd been playing with happily. I'd ask how long he'd protested for. 'Only two minutes.' Well then – why was this a problem? If he'd continued to be upset for more than ten minutes, I would have understood. If Aaron didn't look up at the very moment when someone came into the classroom, then it was because he was 'in his own world' and wasn't being attentive enough to his environment, irrespective of the fact that most of the other kids didn't look up either.

It was clear to me that Aaron was being overly scrutinised. Everything he did was being watched through a magnifying glass.

Aaron's imaginary play was spectacular and he totally disappeared into the scenes he created. After all, we'd taught him imaginary play and he was doing exactly what we'd asked of him. But because he'd engage in imaginary play at school, he was labelled as 'being stuck in his imagination'. When the speech therapist tried to test his language skills, she struggled to get Aaron to remain on topic as he wanted to take her into his jungle scene. Instead of redirecting Aaron to focus on the discussion, as she would do with any other child, she came to the conclusion that he couldn't remain engaged. It was a fait accompli. It would have taken her very little effort to get him back on topic, but as he had been labelled as a kid with a problem, no one was prepared to show him the way.

Learning about school rules

Getting Aaron to sustain his attention in the classroom *was* a hurdle. Luckily, Carolynn's experience often got us through these worrying times. She wasn't concerned about Aaron, and reassured me that he *would* be successful. Once he understood what was expected of him, he'd follow the rules. She was right. As soon as Aaron realised that he had to follow rules at school, he began to sustain his attention.

Before circle time, the facilitator would remind him of these rules. Eyes and body in the group; no imaginary play during circle; no fiddling and no sleeping. Look, listen and pay attention. This worked and eventually we no longer needed to remind Aaron what was expected of him at school. For almost four years, we had created a world that revolved around him. Now he had to learn to wait his turn when he was in a group and transfer the skills we'd taught him to a classroom setting.

During his one-on-one sessions at home in the cottage, we'd reverse the roles. He would be the teacher and his instructors would pretend they weren't listening or started to fiddle while Aaron was telling them a story. He'd have to identify that they were no longer paying attention, and remind them of the rules. This worked very well in getting Aaron to understand what was expected of him at school.

We also paired listening and paying attention in class with a high rein-forcer at the end of the day – mostly that meant going onto YouTube on my computer once he got home. As the weeks passed, Aaron became success-ful at school. He had just needed a foot up.

Another win

Aaron came with a history and therefore the school judged him unfairly. The teachers had no idea where he'd started from: we dug him out from under the rubble. Yet he'd fought so hard – harder than any other child – to earn his place at school. He needed them to believe in him; to teach him in the same way they taught any other child and to have the same expecta-tions of him as they had of the rest of the class. I struggled to find the right words to explain to them that he was catching up. It was so difficult not to sound defensive.

'He can't do it,' the teacher told me, after he'd answered incorrectly dur-ing circle time. The facilitator was there to step in and I realised that we needed to move control over to the teacher. It was time to fade out the facilitator. At the same time, if the teachers were not going to have the same expectations of Aaron as they had of the other kids, we'd struggle to fade her out. This was a very sensitive situation and I agonised over the right course of action. How were we going to get the teachers to believe in Aaron?

In time, I realised that only Aaron held the key. He'd have to prove himself. After four months in Grade R, even though the school still had reservations about Aaron's potential success, we insisted on fading out the facilitator to move control over to the teacher. We knew Aaron was ready, and he proved us right.

An impartial educational-psychology assessment

Aaron no longer went to school with his facilitator. My team would simply do a monthly school visit to check on him and speak to his teacher. As the weeks passed, it became clear that Aaron was becoming more independent and successful at school.

In order for us to secure Aaron's place in mainstream Grade 1, the school requested a school-readiness assessment. The thought of having Aaron assessed by an educational psychologist made me very nervous. Nevertheless, an objective opinion was a good idea and would give Aaron's teacher the reassurance she needed. The assessment was also required if we were to have Aaron officially re-assessed as having 'recovered' from autism.

A few years back, I'd had a bad experience with a speech therapist who had assessed Aaron's language skills. She was familiar with our family history and hadn't given Aaron the opportunity of a fair assessment. This is a common theme once a child receives that learning challenge label. This time, I was determined to ensure an impartial and objective assessment. I did my research and chose an educational psychologist who ticked all my boxes. I'd read a report she'd done on another child: a comprehensive account of the child's skill set. From that I'd been able to tell that she was experienced and paid attention to detail.

The night before my appointment with her I got into bed and turned off the light, only to jump up a few minutes later when it hit me that I hadn't filled in the information she required prior to meeting with a child's parent. Completing the 15-page document was an interesting exercise. I wanted an unbiased opinion and was determined to get one. The next step was an hour's meeting with her, going over the reasons why I wanted the assessment and discussing Aaron. I was very careful not to give away who I was – nor did I disclose that Aaron had a brother with autism. She concluded that I was an anxious parent and offered to do parent training for me after the assessment. I couldn't help but giggle. She had no idea where we'd come from and the terrain we'd covered before arriving at her door. It was within my discretion whether to grant permission for his teacher to discuss the report with her. I chose to bypass Aaron's teacher. This meant that the psychologist's assessment of Aaron wouldn't be influenced by the teacher's description of his performance in class; and that he was afforded the opportunity of an impartial assessment – something that isn't always possible.

The purpose of the educational psychologist's assessment was to give an indication of Aaron's current level of ability and possible areas of strength and weakness. The tests administered included the:

❏ Wechsler Preschool and Primary Scale of Intelligence, Fourth Edition (WPPSI IV)
❏ Junior South African Individual Scale (JSAIS) – Story Memory Subtest; Draw a Person [DAP]; Colour a Person [CAP]; and
❏ Bender Visual-Motor Gestalt Test, Second Edition (Bender II)
❏ Perceptual-Assessment Tool; Curriculum-Based Assessment (CBA)
❏ Kindergarten Readiness Test (KRT)

The purpose of the above tests would be to measure Aaron's cognition, sensory-motor skills, social and emotional maturity, and cognitive and academic skills. He was assessed over two days. I sat outside in the car waiting for him. The psychologist didn't give away how he'd performed and I waited anxiously for our next meeting, when she would disclose the results. I insisted on taking my own detailed notes during her feedback session, as this would be invaluable when I gave feedback to Carolynn.

Words we never thought we'd hear
The educational psychologist's report concluded:

> *Aaron is a delightful and engaging little boy and he entered the assessment room happily. Rapport was quickly established and Aaron made*

eye contact and was able to engage easily in conversation, demonstrating age-appropriate social skills.

According to the results from the WPPSI IV Aaron scored in the average range for the Verbal Comprehension Index, Processing Speed Index, Fluid Reasoning Index, Visual Spatial Index and Working Memory Index. Aaron's full-scale IQ fell in the average range.

Aaron has a very good knowledge of concepts. He enjoys learning new things and it's evident that learning is taking place. Aaron is school ready and should be able to manage a formal Grade 1 curriculum next year.

There was no mention of autism or anything close to it. We had succeeded in defeating autism! Some parents might be disappointed to hear their child's IQ isn't on the genius scale, but we'd worked so hard with Aaron that just hearing he was 'average' was music to our ears and a huge victory.

I sent Carolynn a copy of the report and eagerly awaited her comments. She came back immediately: 'I read the report ... I have to hold back tears. Amazing. He did it. I want to frame the sentence "Rapport was quickly established and Aaron made eye contact and was able to engage easily in conversation, demonstrating age-appropriate social skills." That is gold!!! I'm just so happy for you and Martin I can't put it into words – I knew he could do it. You have so much to celebrate.'

Aaron starts big school (Grade 1)

Like any child about to start 'big school', Aaron was beyond excited. He'd gotten out his new school bag and lunch box a dozen times, giving me instructions as to what should go into each. It was clear he was thrilled to be embarking on this new adventure and chapter in his life. This was a day that Martin and I had thought we'd never see, and we too were delighted and caught up in the excitement.

Eventually, Aaron went to bed and fell asleep dreaming about the next day – his first day of 'big school'. I sat on the edge of his bed and studied his angelic face as he slept peacefully. The new addition to his toy collection, a big green triceratops we'd bought at the toy shop

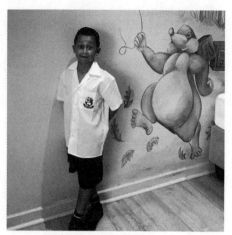

Aaron in Grade 1

earlier that day, was tucked safely under his arm. His *The Lion King* set, including his two favourite characters Simba and Nala, lay at the foot of his bed. He'd been playing with them, acting out a scene from the movie, before eventually agreeing to climb into bed. It had taken much negotiation before he'd accepted the good night deal I'd proposed. We'd agreed on 20 animal 'I spy's", 20 kisses and two stories before I turned off the light.

'Mom, why do I have to go to bed?' he asked me as I wrestled him to sleep.

'Because tomorrow is a big day and you need your rest,' I replied as I kissed his forehead.

'Hold my hand, Mom,' he requested as he snuggled closer to me. 'I love you Mom,' he said as he turned over just before falling asleep. I'll never tire of hearing those three words from Aaron. Words I have so desperately wished for – but never heard – from David.

Rocco, our chocolate Labrador, jumped onto the bed and took his place next to Aaron as he did every night, guarding over him as he slept. Rocco's face was buried in the duvet, but his big brown paw remained on Aaron's leg. Aaron and Rocco are best friends and share a special connection. Aaron had included Rocco in his *The Lion King* scene earlier, running down the corridor with a biscuit as Rocco charged behind him trying to grab the biscuit and creating a stampede. Rocco represented the wildebeest in *The Lion King* …

Earlier that day, Aaron had helped me label his stationery. We packed his crayons and oil pencils into his black Mickey Mouse pencil case, a gift from Jacky. Aaron particularly adored elephants and a family of elephants stood on the shelf in his room. So naturally, when he was choosing a new school bag, there was only one choice – an orange elephant bag.

I'd already laid out his school clothes in preparation for the next day. His new black school shoes – shiny and polished – lay on the floor waiting to be worn. As I turned to go, I looked at the candle that was standing on the mantlepiece flickering in the dark, its warm glow creating a shadow on the ceiling, a reminder that Aaron was a miracle. We had lit the candle in the earliest, darkest days of our journey with Aaron's autism as a manifestation of hope and light; and it was now burning brightly as it does every night, representing our victory over the disease.

Aaron woke early the next morning to get ready for school. He hurried to the breakfast table bustling with excitement and jabbering on about what he'd planned for the day. 'Don't forget to pack celery for my snack, Mom,' he reminded me. Aaron's favourite snack was celery, carrots and cucumber, as he'd learnt from a very young age to eat vegetables and healthy snacks. I arrived at the table as I had for the past four years, with a bunch of medications for him to swallow. Breakfast was scrambled eggs and tomato and Aaron hungrily ate his food. 'Mom,' he reminded me, 'you forgot my nose spray.' I hurried over to the corner of my kitchen where I kept all his medicines and found the nose spray. 'No injection today, Mom,' he told me as he took another mouthful of his scrambled eggs.

'No injection today Aaron – that will only be on Friday.'

'Is Jacky taking me to school today?' he asked.

'Not today,' I replied. 'You're going on your own, just like a big boy.'

How privileged I felt to be a part of Aaron's first day of big school! He clutched my hand tightly as we walked to his new classroom and I was bursting with pride as we entered the room. His friend Joshua came running over to Aaron, grabbed his hand and led him to a group of boys who were playing on the floor mat. As Aaron confidently joined their game, I waved goodbye and turned to leave.

However, I was feeling just a little protective. 'Don't forget to listen out for the school bell,' I couldn't help yelling across the room before I made my exit.

Life today with Aaron

Aaron has lost his diagnosis of autism. He can tell us what he's thinking and where he wants to go, what he likes and doesn't like, and just like any other little boy his age, he enjoys play dates, sleepovers at granny's house and going to the movies. We got our boy back. We won the battle.

Not so with our first son David, who continues to be imprisoned in a physical body that has partly succumbed to the wounds inflicted upon him by his autism. Yet it is David who, in large part, was responsible for saving his brother: what we learnt in trying to save David paved the way for most of the treatments that ultimately led to Aaron's recovery.

HOME FREE

Aaron looks forward to our regular trips to the park with our dogs Rocco and Miley. He continues to surprise us and creeps into the hearts of all those who come across his path. Since he has full functionality, he's been given a second chance to live a full life. Sometimes I have to remind myself that his autism really did happen, as it seems so unreal. Aaron found his way out of the darkness and into the light. No longer lost in the woods, he is home safe.

Aaron is a happy boy who loves life itself, a miracle child who proved that autism is in fact *something children can recover from*. As I think about the path we've walked, I'm reminded of conversations with Aaron I haven't had to miss; and of the joy of being able to hear him sing his songs. There are so many things to be glad and relieved about.

Hearing his voice when I wake up in the morning and knowing whether he's happy, sore or sad, because he can tell me how he's feeling. Searching the house with him to help him find one of his lost toys. Savouring every moment of watching him graduate from nursery to big school. Celebrating his birthday and choosing his cake and the theme for his birthday party. Playing 'I Spy with my Little Eye' and reading him stories as he rests his head on my shoulder. Trying to solve his problems, which include not being able to take the dogs with him on holiday, and entails answering thousands of questions. Hearing the screams and laughter of his pillow fights with Eli fill the house and knowing his favourite colour and what he likes to eat. Watching when he gets a surprise or hearing his expression of delight when he bites into a warm slice of pizza. Taking him to the zoo and the farm and sharing in his interest and love of animals. Hearing him tell me he loves me and watching him call out 'Daddy' as he runs down the passage to greet Martin when he arrives back home from work. Taking him to soccer and karate …

All of this has been wonderful and we've enjoyed and treasured every single minute of it. Even though it took four long years of an ABA programme, brave medical treatments, sacrifice, blood, sweat and tears, it was all worth it and I would do it all over again in a heartbeat.

Martin, Aaron and I regularly make what we call a 'sandwich' on our bed, where Martin and I are the bread and Aaron gets to choose which filling he wants to be as all three of us squash together tight. Aaron receives an outpouring of affection. I don't think a day goes by in which we don't hug and squeeze him to pieces.

When light dispels darkness

During the Jewish festival of Hanukkah, I'm reminded of our victorious battle with autism. Hanukkah is an eight-day 'festival of lights', celebrated with nightly candle-lighting and special prayers. The word 'Hanukkah' means 'dedication'; and the festival celebrates the re-dedication of the Second Temple in Jerusalem. It is also linked to the story that, after the destruction of the Second Temple, the one-day supply of oil to light the candelabra miraculously lasted for eight nights.

Each night we light the candelabra. One candle for each of the eight nights, until on the final night, all eight candles shine brightly. As the number of candles increases each night, there is more light available to dispel the darkness. The physical act of lighting the candles teaches us we're all like a candle burning, dispelling darkness in our lives and in the world.

We witness miracles every day and may sometimes take them for granted. However, Martin and I never took Aaron's progress and development for granted. He was a miracle and we were well aware of this. We savoured every single moment of him and he brought light into our home and our lives.

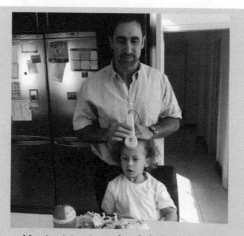

Martin giving Aaron low-light laser therapy

How did I feel when we started to realise there were signs Aaron wasn't developing as he should be? After all, we'd just watched ten years of the David movie. The movie of autism. And when you've watched a movie like that you know what's going to happen. And when you've seen your first child deteriorate, battle and regress over ten years and suddenly you're faced with another child going down the same path, it's extremely frightening. Facing a whole new world of worry you can't describe is paralysing and you end up not knowing what to do.

Many parents know what it is to have their child go out at night and worry until they're home and safely tucked in bed. But once they're tucked up the worry goes away – at least for now. With Aaron, that worry was indefinite. It was there all the time. Will he be like David? Will we be able to save him? That was our constant companion – worry. When we went to bed at night, and woke in the morning – it just consumed us.

Denial

At the beginning we'd try and reassure ourselves that it wasn't so bad – it was just a phase he was going through. It's difficult to put our feelings into words over such a long period of time. It wasn't minutes, hours, days or weeks. It unfolded over months. So from one day to the next, if he had a good day then we'd be okay. Then he'd be almost okay and we'd convince ourselves he was fine and that we'd been over-analysing. From having a child like David, analysing everything was second nature to us.

Eventually we came to a point where things changed. We turned from people who were paralysed and hoping this wasn't what we'd thought it was, to one day deciding: this is a problem and now we're going to deal with it. Suddenly everything felt so much better. Worrying about something is always worse than the thing itself.

Critical action

I say we, but it was very much all Ilana, with me in the supporting role. She was in the thick of things. And after ten years of dealing with David and never giving up, always fighting at full strength and not, as I expected, getting burnt out, now she had to raise her game completely and fight for two kids. If she was ever going to burn out it was now. But she didn't! She kept on fighting and dug very, very deep to save Aaron. She analysed every bit of his programme, making sure he achieved all his goals on time.

In every sport or discipline there's always the expert, the best in the world, the person who's more skilled than anyone else. The tennis player with his precise shots – absolute perfection to watch. When he wins, he's playing against the best in the world. There are millions of people who have practised tennis over and over again, trying to qualify for competitions, going through rounds of opponents before they get to the top. So when you get to that level, every inch of your game has to be perfect. At that point in time, Ilana was at the top of her game. She was the best at what she needed to do and it was out of a pure life or death situation. She had to be a skilled tightrope walker, and if she fell it would be to her death. She had no choice but to make it to the other side. That's how she fought this fight.

It was working …

She lived and breathed Aaron's war, even more than she'd done with David, using all the knowledge she'd gathered over the years of David's ABA programme. But the biggest motivating factor was the progress Aaron made, unlike that of any other child we'd ever seen before. Whatever medication we gave him seemed to help. Whatever ABA we used, it worked. It was by no means easy going but you could see the progress.

Of course, there were also many times when he just stagnated and we'd bang our heads against the wall. We were consumed with Aaron's progress and didn't talk about anything else.

There was no normal conversation around the dinner table, discussing friends, family or other things. It was 80 per cent Aaron and 20 per cent David. Sadly, with no space for Eli. We had to talk about Aaron or drown. Other topics were meaningless right then. There were times when I thought that maybe our life could have been so different and now we had to go through this again. But the main difference between this experience and dealing with David is that this time I didn't feel sorry for myself. With David I was upset and angry, and couldn't believe such a thing could happen to anybody. With Aaron it wasn't really like that. I was over that. Now I just had to deal with it.

Finding the key

We were just so lucky Aaron made the progress he did, which is very rare. ABA definitely works – Aaron's proof of this. The main principle was to find ways of motivating him to do what we wanted him to do. Time and again Ilana would unlock the puzzle, buy new material, and try different approaches, which worked. That feeling of success was indescribable. All the tiny steps to all those little gains made the difference.

Unlocking his voice

The many months when Aaron didn't speak at all were extremely worrying. Again, we knew what this meant – having had David nonverbal for so many years, frustrated at not being able to communicate his needs. So for Aaron to be silent was a very scary place to be and unfortunately no matter how much you try and how much ABA you use, you just never know whether you'll get your child to speak. You wonder if maybe your child's brain isn't wired to generate that voice production. One speech therapist said they didn't think he'd speak very well – if at all. Ilana took an apraxic child who should never have spoken and got him to speak. It was an absolute miracle.

When he said his first few words, we felt this enormous weight slowly lifting off our shoulders. It was incredible. Each and every word was so precious and meant so much. Each sound was like a birthday celebration and we didn't take anything for granted. Even now that Aaron is six and has spoken for a long time, we still bask in everything he says. We cherish and love him so much.

The sunshine kid

Aaron nowadays is such a happy boy. Looking back, he actually loved his years of ABA and all the attention he got. He loved playing with his toys and the interaction with his therapists. So, to those people who say ABA is destructive and repetitive and just creates robots, that's complete rubbish! If ABA is done in the correct way, the child can be motivated and absolutely love it.

I so enjoy taking him to school in the morning: he leaves home with a spring in his step, always smiling and enjoying life. He loves all his toys and the gifts he receives. He cherishes them all and is just happy to be Aaron. We get so much joy from this child with his cute sense of humour. There's no way to adequately express our love for him. Not a day or even a minute goes by when we don't appreciate the miracle that is Aaron.

Hope and will win every time

There are a few key words to this story. One is 'hope', but greater than that is the word 'will'. If somebody wills something that much, it will happen. If you're on a deserted island and you know you need to survive and have the will to survive, then you will. You'll find water, a coconut – something to keep you going. You'll work out how to live and survive – if you want to. If you give up hope by imagining that no one is coming to fetch you and you're going to die there, you'll lose the will to live and you'll die. Ilana had the strongest will of anyone I know. She was determined and willed Aaron to win his fight. She wouldn't give up, which was crucial to our success in healing Aaron.

Hope is a lesser form of will, but just as important. As long as hope is there, you can keep will alive. You always have to have hope and look at the positive in everything – no matter how bad it seems. If you can see some light around the next corner you can carry on going in the right direction, but the second you lose hope you're finished.

This means you have to find ways of keeping that hope alive. That's the best advice I can give any parent. When you're trying new medications, if one doesn't work, try another. If you've tried an ABA technique and it didn't work, move on to the next one. If you tried a motivator and that didn't work – look for another one to replace it. There's always something else. Keep hope alive and you'll succeed.

CHAPTER TWENTY-TWO

ELI'S STORY

Eli is the only one of our children to have escaped a diagnosis of autism. Of course, this doesn't mean that he has been left untouched by the disease. All our lives have been ruled by autism to a greater or lesser degree. Consumed by his siblings' next treatment or therapy session, Eli simply had to grow up fast.

Raising Eli and experiencing the normal joys of parenting got us through exceptionally treacherous times. If we hadn't had Eli to take our minds off autism, we'd certainly have gone mad. He helped normalise our lives and

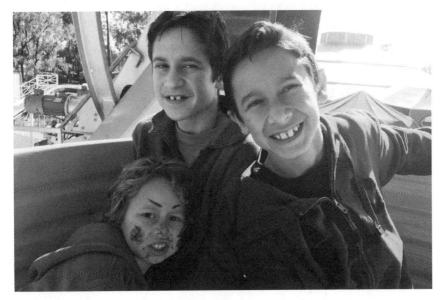

David, Eli and Aaron

was a deviation from our sorrow. There was no better medicine than getting lost in Eli's world for a brief moment, to soothe the pain we'd been experiencing with another day of trying to help David or a very young Aaron. Dropping him at a normal school was a treat.

I sobbed at every single one of his school concerts. Eventually I was struggling to attend them, as I inevitably drew attention to myself, causing quite the scene with my puffy red eyes. Tears flowed freely from my face while I tried desperately to turn off the waterworks. Every time I went to one of his concerts, I felt numb. I cried for so many reasons. Tears of sadness for all the concerts David would never be a part of. Tears of gratitude that Eli had made it in one piece – autism free. It was bitter-sweet.

Making the milestones

Eli's language developed on time. He was in fact advanced for his age. He spoke with ease. There was no fussing over Eli. He was the perfect child born to parents preoccupied with a war on autism. If he cried, I took absolutely no notice; and he learnt early on that he was expected to speak and use his words to get his message across.

During primary school, his teachers would always praise him – 'easy kid', 'clever kid', 'follows instructions', 'diligent student' and 'well-liked by his peers'. Their comments also included 'Tends to talk a lot.' If Eli ever got into trouble at school, it was for asking *too many* questions. He was the kind of kid who sailed through school – a model student. But Eli is also a kind, caring soul who learnt early on that the world is much less than perfect. He has experienced brokenness and sadness more than most other children his age.

Uncle Alan fills some gaps

Martin's brother Alan played a supportive role in Eli's life in the early years. Uncle Alan would spend time with Eli, playing with him or taking him out for a milkshake. This alleviated our feelings of guilt about being controlled by autism. Eli deserved a life outside of autism and Uncle Alan gave him that. What mattered was that he was getting time away from the disease that held us captive. Time to simply enjoy the moment and take it all in, without having his time controlled by David's tantrums. We never took Eli to the zoo or made a trip with him to the local fire station, and so missed out on seeing the look on his face when he experienced these things.

Even though Eli was born second, in many ways he's regarded as the eldest child and has taken on the responsibility of what that means. We've tried to prepare him for the future in ways that are realistic but neither overwhelming nor unfair.

Just the other day he asked me: 'Mom, if you and Dad die together, must David live with me in my house?'

'No, Eli – you'll live with *your* family … But you'll be the one to see to his well-being. This means you'll need to manage the people David lives with, to ensure that the highest standard of care is provided for him.'

Quite a large responsibility for a 13-year-old to comprehend!

An understanding beyond his years

Countless times, I've stood next to Eli in a public place or at a grocery store when David has had a tantrum and caused a terrible scene. Eli's calm and tolerant attitude towards David has surprised me each time. Never once has he gotten angry or blamed David for his outbursts. He's been as annoyed as I have, and we may have voiced this once we were safely back in the car, but I've never heard him say how unpleasant it is for him or that he hates David for it. Eli has felt embarrassed and it hasn't made him feel good to see his brother so distressed – but he has never blamed David.

A de facto guardian over his brothers, he finds himself babysitting them regularly. I'll leave him with the phone in his hand and, as I'm about to escape out the door, we'll go over the emergency plan. 'First call the ambulance and then me,' I remind him as I fly out the door to do my chores so that I can race back as fast as I can. Eli has basic training in first aid as I've tried to equip him for any eventuality, especially since David sometimes suffers from seizures.

Growing up with a brother like David has moulded his personality, and he sees the world differently from the ways in which many more carefree 13-year-old teenagers view it.

Eli's take on autism, his brother David and life in general

Being David's brother is harder than people would ever imagine. I've always wanted to have an older brother that would be there to stick up for me, guide me and teach me skills I never had. You can get lonely not having anyone to talk to, especially with your parents being very busy most of the time.

Other kids are very lucky to have a brother or sister who can always keep them company. For me this hasn't been the case – I wasn't as lucky. It's very difficult for a seven-year-old to see his older brother have a tantrum in the shopping mall or in public places. I've had to adapt and learn, and try to understand why David acts like this. I know that I'll always be the one who has to look out for him.

I know David inside out. When I was little, I thought he'd just speak like we all do. As I grew older, I realised how hard it was for him to produce words and express himself. I also miss not having an older brother who can play games or soccer with me. With this missing part of my life I had to find other friends – and I usually spend my Saturdays either having friends over to our place or going to a friend's house.

A DIFFERENT LIFE

Going on holidays, for instance, is never straightforward. Once we were going on holiday to Umhlanga and I was really excited, but the good time I thought we'd have turned into chaos because we couldn't step out of our apartment without David having a meltdown. It was like living in solitary confinement. When you're just seven years old, watching your brother having a tantrum can affect you in various ways. It upset me and made me feel horrible. To see a human being who happens to be your brother in such a state was devastating.

There was a very bad period when I couldn't remember a single day when David didn't hit his head, scream or wring his nose until it was blue. I would come home from school each day and ask my mom: 'What did David do today?' only to find out they had both had a hard time.

Gradually it became difficult to have friends over to my house. I remember how, a few years ago, a friend was visiting me and we were jumping on the trampoline. David was climbing up the jungle gym and I was having a great time playing with my friend. Suddenly, I see my older brother walk to the middle of the garden, pull down his pants and start peeing on the lawn. While this would be okay if he was five years old, at his age this was not socially acceptable and I was so embarrassed I wanted to curl up in a ball and cry. As embarrassed as I was, though, I asked my friend to turn around and close his eyes. When David walked away, my friend suggested I should just tell him not to do it again. How could I explain to my friend I didn't think it was going to be that simple for David?

I can remember going to a Pick 'n Pay shopping centre. We were shopping as usual and David's anxiety was building. Every time we went shopping it was as if we were walking next to a mobile time bomb. When the time ran out, it would set off the bomb. And this wasn't a pretty sight. To see David shriek, all you wanted to do was hide away behind your mom and hope no one you knew could see you.

Now I'm older I realise that as much as I used to hide behind my mom, my mom has no one to hide behind and has had to deal with the stares and burning glares of utter disbelief we've had from other people. It always angered me how people didn't have the decency to look away and save us from the embarrassment. But unfortunately, society was insensitive to us.

BEING THE BEST I COULD BE

I thought that things might get better and that it couldn't get any worse. I was wrong. The older I got the more aware I became and the more I realised how bad the situation really was with David. As a young kid you're less aware. I had to grow up faster because I had to be responsible and I knew that I couldn't cause my parents any more dread, so I tried to study hard and be a diligent student and make up for what David didn't give them. It was enough for my parents to have to deal with David. I didn't want to disappoint my parents and add to their burden. So I always tried extra hard at school to give them a little bit of pleasure in their life. I could see how hard my parents worked every day to take care of David's needs and I didn't want to add to their troubles.

Autism and The Star Academy have been a popular topic of conversation in our house for many years. As a younger kid I used to ask my parents if they could please talk about something else. I will admit there were times where I felt deprived of attention. My parents were constantly involved in David's needs and when Aaron arrived on the scene it became even worse as I slipped to the very bottom of their attention list. This was another reason that drove me to do well academically, because I wanted more of their attention – and the way to get it was to be successful at school. Kids who crave attention usually get themselves into trouble to get their parents to notice them. I couldn't do that as it would have broken my parents.

AUTISM ISN'T WHAT PEOPLE THINK!
My school friends have never understood what autism means and what it's like living with David. It infuriates me when I see movies or videos or people saying that people with autism see the world differently and are just socially odd. And that we mustn't move them out of their world into ours. This is the furthest thing from the truth anyone could ever say. What autism really is about is being unable to function as a human being. Not only do people with autism not see the world differently, they don't see the world at all. Autism is people who scream and tantrum and inflict pain on themselves. Autism is a family's worst nightmare. Society doesn't want to see autistic people for who they really are.

When I was younger, I used to wonder how David knew how to

type words and the alphabet, yet couldn't speak. To this day I still wonder about that. When we were first introduced to the Dynavox I thought it was the coolest piece of machinery I'd ever laid eyes on. To me it was David's thought translator – just as in the movie *Cloudy with a Chance of Meatballs*, where the monkey has a thought translator and the device says everything he's thinking. Today David uses his iPad to ask us questions. These questions are programmed for him to get information. He often asks questions about what he'll be doing at school or when he'll be going on a certain outing to the BOUNCE trampoline park or Acrobranch. David becomes anxious if we don't answer him and so we make an effort to give him the information he needs.

I often watch my brothers if my parents have important meetings to go to or if they're Skyping with America. I feel a responsibility to act as the older brother and supervise them.

Have you ever had one of those days where you wake up to a wonderful day, the sun is streaming in, the birds are chirping and you feel great? Unfortunately for our family, many times we've had to wake up to the sounds of David's horrific screaming and banging his head against the wall at 5 am. Many times before going to bed, instead of saying good night to my parents and brothers I'd have to go to my room to escape David's screaming and then fall asleep with a heavy heart.

GETTING THROUGH THE TOUGH TIMES

I try not to think about David's situation and every time David's going through a good patch I think to myself that it isn't so bad – but the cracks start creeping in and the monster called autism appears again, popping its head in and challenging us.

David had been ill for a few days and wasn't getting any better. I remember playing Nintendo in my room when I was suddenly interrupted by my parents and told to pack my bags. David was to be admitted to hospital and I was going to spend the night at my Uncle Alan. This was just one of many times when I had to be brave.

I used to feel that autism was the end of the world. Over time, I realised we could still be a happy family and live with it. We often go to the Vaal River where we keep a boat and my dad pulls us down the river on a tube. I sit next to David on the tube and as much as I enjoy flying through the water, I always feel concerned about David flipping over. I feel responsible for him all the time.

ADJUSTING YOUR LIFE TO SEIZURES

I do think about all the things we lost – like David not having a bar mitzvah. When I was little, I used to think we'd programme his Dynavox to say the bar mitzvah speech for him, but as I got older I realised this wasn't going to happen. I never got to make a speech at his bar mitzvah or hear his friends talk about what a special friend he is. I didn't have an older brother whose friends included me in their group or who could teach me how to play soccer.

David went through a phase when he broke absolutely everything he could lay his hands on and I've lost many valuable items that were special to me that way, from my sunglasses to my bag to my books and even my clothes.

I feel terrible that David has to take so many medicines every day and it's not pleasant to take the ones that taste horrible or are big and hard to swallow. I feel really sorry he has to need all these medicines to keep his tantrums at bay. He has to take seizure medication; and it's always a worry that he could have a seizure at any moment.

I remember the first time David had a seizure. I was at school and when I got home, instead of having my mom tell me about her day, I had to learn that my brother had had a seizure. It made me feel very worried that he might die and it added even more responsibility because I had to learn what to do in case of a seizure. The second time it happened, I was at home and had a friend over to play. We were playing Lego when we were interrupted by David falling off the chair in the dining room. My mom had to call the ambulance. I told my friend to wait in the kitchen with me until the ambulance arrived. After this incident I'd often wake up in a sweat, having had a nightmare about David having a seizure.

David has even had a seizure on a plane. I was sitting next to him and, as we landed, I felt relieved to be on the ground. The relief was short-lived because, as I turned, I saw my brother shaking uncontrollably with his eyes rolled back. All eyes were on us and one of the passengers on the plane asked if he was okay. I wished she hadn't because, duh – did he look okay? She was just being nosy. Many people stared as David was wheeled off the plane. Instead of being excited to get back home, we took some time to get over this. The seizures are always a shock. It feels like when you walk into a room and someone hiding behind the door shouts, 'Boo!' You don't quite get over David having a seizure.

And then there was the incident at my grandmother's house where my grandmother and I thought he'd died. I was scarred for life.

HE AIN'T HEAVY, HE'S MY BROTHER

Even though David has autism and life can be hard with him, I still love him and wouldn't want anything bad to ever happen to him. He has taught me to appreciate life and being able to function properly. I never take for granted things I can do easily that he's unable to do, like being able to have friends or communicate my needs and have a conversation. I still hold on to the hope that David will continue to recover from autism and live a happy life. I've become used to David's limitations and have created my own world within these limitations. My expectations are different. David has taught me to be responsible and not to take anything for granted, as life is fragile.

My tips for siblings of autistic children are:

1. Don't get angry with your brother or sister because they can't help being irritating and annoying sometimes.
2. When your brother or sister with autism has a meltdown in public, stare directly back at the people looking at you in utter shock. They'll look away in no time.
3. Don't get angry if your brother or sister doesn't understand your instruction. Break it down into small steps and keep your language simple.

4. True friends are those who accept you have a sibling with challenges and don't judge you for it.
5. Don't ever give up hope, because there are many ways to help autistic children lead better lives.
6. Try to help your parents in any small way you can. They're having a hard time dealing with autism.
7. Enjoy your life. Don't let autism pull you down. Celebrate the special moments and know that things will get better.

The miracle that is Eli

When Eli was little, I'd often feel exhausted and defeated by autism. Our collision with the disease uncovered a part of me that I hated, but I had no choice. I had to keep going. I had to become a fortress, burying my emotions in a place where even I couldn't reach them. There were days when autism made me unkind and impatient, and looking back it sometimes feels to me as if there *was* a chapter in time when Eli was exposed to a cold mother – one who was devoid of any emotion.

During the early stages of his development, I was wrestling with great fear. A topic constantly on my mind was whether he would develop normally. Not only did we have to deal with David's illness, but we also had to make sure to take great care around anything and everything Eli came into contact with. By then we knew there were environmental triggers for autism, and protecting Eli against them weighed heavily on our shoulders. We did our research and consulted the experts, but in the end we had to reach our own conclusions. This took a great deal of energy and bravery.

I became rock-hard – an impenetrable fortress. In no time, the only way I could cope was to run an army base. I was all business, every minute of every day. Although I realised that I was struggling to engage and play with Eli, I couldn't let my guard down to have fun with him. I was simply too sad, and in too much pain. Martin was just the opposite, luckily. He could relax and play with Eli, and they enjoyed many content and fun moments together.

In time, however, Eli managed to bring me around with his gentle and caring nature. His attractive character and infectiously happy attitude infiltrated the house and brightened my world. I began to allow myself to let him into my heart. His sweet voice eventually sealed the deep void there. His cute comments and insistence on getting my attention started to penetrate the wall I'd built around my emotions and I developed a deep love for my little boy. He'd gaze up at me with his deep, penetrating brown eyes and I'd melt instantly.

Eli could communicate with ease and confidence from the start, which was a huge relief and brought us endless happiness. When we heard him put together increasingly complicated sentences, we knew we'd managed to save him from a world of isolation in which being able to express oneself verbally is an immense struggle. We had avoided having to fight – and maybe lose – a terrifying battle!

I could not wait to fetch him from school and hear all about his day. Taking Eli to the toyshop was another real treat. 'Mommy, I want the green train,' he'd effortlessly request while pointing towards the object of his desire. It was hard to resist buying him absolutely everything he asked for!

Bustling about determinedly with bits of news and information, he brought variety and joy into our lives. His many stories and interesting titbits added fuel to our petrol tanks, which had been running on empty before his arrival on the scene. His enthusiasm for everything around him became medicine for my soul, and I started to heal from all the pain and bitterness.

He was a confident and fluent reader from a very young age, and we'd often find him buried in his books. Eli caught on quickly to new facts and ideas. He was also enthusiastic about learning and as his school career advanced his certificates of merit for excellence poured in. His desire to please and his wonderful achievements lifted our spirits.

From early on, Eli displayed a strongly moral approach to life. He has deep-rooted beliefs and convictions coupled with high intelligence. Thanks to his strong sense of right and wrong, we have always been able to rely on him for great behaviour. When Eli went to a friend's house or came into contact with another adult, without fail we'd receive approving reports on his behaviour and impeccable manners. This made us feel extremely proud and gave us a sense of accomplishment as parents.

Already perceptive as a little boy, Eli has retained his deeper under-standing of human nature. The one constant in our life, he's been patient with both his brothers and – most of all – his parents, who continue to jug-gle demanding circumstances. He is very proud of the achievements David has made along the way and is willing to defend him even at substantial cost to himself. As a result of all these qualities, all the memories we have of Eli and his role in our life are cherished ones.

We know Eli will do something astounding with his life. He has all the ingredients for success. Our love for him runs very deep and we continue to draw a great deal of comfort knowing he is here.

Not a single day goes by when we don't acknowledge the miracle that is Eli.

CHAPTER TWENTY-THREE

THE ROAD TO RECOVERY: CLOSING THOUGHTS

That diagnosed autism is a condition for which children can be treated – and from which many of them can recover to various degrees or even entirely – was already known in 1987. In that year, Dr Ole Ivar Lovaas published the results of his groundbreaking study on the use of ABA in treating children with autism. The children he had studied were between three and four years old, and had received seven hours of ABA a day. The study proved a 47 per cent recovery rate from autism. No wonder he became a hero to so many parents!

Keeping hope alive

No one will deny that the devastation of the experience of autism can result in the loss of hope. Every day is a physical and emotional slog as one works towards achieving set goals. Hitting a brick wall trying to save David was a regular occurrence for us. It was incredibly difficult not to lose all hope, especially when we'd invested so much time, effort and money in his treatments. This type of outlay – heavy in every way – inevitably sets up expectations. When these aren't fulfilled and your whole world collapses, it's a challenge to believe that things will eventually work out.

The more we focused on the negatives, however, the deeper we dug a dark hole for ourselves. In time, we learnt that finding the positives and staying focused on the blessings in our lives helped us to escape the gloom and despair attached to the negatives.

It was the things we could have taken for granted each day that we made a conscious decision to acknowledge; I'd say them out loud and take a moment to really think about the fact that I had a roof over my head, food to feed my family, a supportive husband, my health, and so on. Having access to the true experts in the field of autism and being guided by them was certainly also instrumental in keeping my hope alive.

Because we had to push through the hurt and pain time and time again, however, it was natural that we should feel discouraged at times. Tackling the long list of endless problems autism presented wasn't easy. Yet keeping a perspective on things and unravelling each stumbling block until we found a way to fight back always kept our hope alive.

Hope implies a certain amount of perseverance, such as believing that a positive outcome is possible even when there's strong evidence to the contrary. As time wore on and David got older without making all the improvements we'd hoped for, we did feel our hope slipping away and scrambled to keep our fear and anxiety in check. Although a voice inside me reminded me of the complexities of our circumstances, I kept on hoping. This despite mounting evidence that David wasn't turning the corner or making his way out of the woods.

We still hoped to get to discover his voice; do those things 'typical' families do, like going to a restaurant or window-shopping at the mall; witness his growing understanding of the world around him; and hear him express himself effortlessly. Above all, we carried on hoping that we would eventually stop seeing him so angry, self-injurious and destructive.

For many years we clung to the hope that he'd feel better and wouldn't have to experience the physical pain we knew he suffered from, including tummy pain, nausea, headaches, dizziness and feelings of discomfort. We held onto hope even when the obstacles we faced seemed insurmountable. There was simply no choice. Giving in to autism was never an option. We were determined in our resolve to find a way, to keep fighting even though we got knocked down by autism countless times. Every knock hurt like hell but we got up and fought back.

There were times when we felt as if autism were a sharp blade placed on our neck, waiting for us to make a false move so it could cause our instant death. There were also many moments when I wondered how we would manage to survive even one more day of that kind of life. Holding on to the belief that we'd be saved, no matter how bad things appeared, was powerful.

Beating autism

When I cast my mind back to the early days of David's diagnosis, I clearly remember the sick feelings of horror and pain we encountered. The fear then of an unknown future and worry of what would become of him and us caused us a deep sense of pain and suffering coupled with grief. The conflict between the inner voice in my heart and my logical mind was a regular occurrence. I'd find myself bargaining with autism in the wee hours of the morning, sleep deprived and not thinking straight as my emotions clouded my intellect. I would draw on my inner strength to pull myself out of the deepest of dark days where hope was a mere flicker in the very far distance.

Looking back now – we made it. We didn't allow autism to prevail. We didn't give in to the overpowering force that stole David from us, leaving him with a physical body that failed him and stripped him of functionality. We always fought back. Autism has been like a magnet clinging to him with a powerful force. Over and over again, we've tried to break the spell. How I wish we could wave a magic wand to make his autism vanish into the air – gone, leaving no trace.

Keeping our hope alive during the hardest days of our lives has only made us stronger. Sometimes I think it's made us too strong …

Even though we were faced with unthinkable hardships, we didn't surrender. Being strong was the only choice we had, even though there were many days when it was tempting to give up. We could choose to let panic and fear overtake us, or we could choose to rise above all the negative feelings we constantly wrestled with. In the best interests of our children we chose to fight for them. For a healthier life – for a good life.

Reflecting on our journey, I'm reminded of all the blessings along the way; and of the many people we met who dedicated – and continue to dedicate – their lives to alleviating the devastation of autism. The doctors who opened their hearts and minds to finding solutions. Those experts we benefited from directly and who kept our hope alive: Dr Granpeesheh, Carolynn Bredyck, Dr Bradstreet and other experts from the United States. Even today, I feel a sense of comfort knowing there are scientists (neurologists, immunologists) from such renowned institutions as Harvard University researching new ways to treat autism. I have no doubt that eventually we will find the cure.

Whether it will be in our lifetime, I can't be sure. But knowing that we have medical professionals such as Dr Granpeesheh and other people dedicating their life's work to the treatment of autism keeps my hope alive.

Recovery from autism (as redefined by Dr Doreen Granpeesheh)

Thinking about recovery can evoke a great deal of emotion. If you're a parent and don't believe that some individuals with autism have the ability to recover 100 per cent, do more research. Open your mind to possibility. Recovered children are no different from any other children. Just because you haven't seen recovery as a professional or a parent, it doesn't mean it doesn't exist.

If recovery from autism weren't possible, medical insurance in the United States wouldn't cover ABA. Insurance funding in the States is granted for what's called 'medical necessity', which means a life-or-death situation. It's not about opinion. There is a great deal of published evidence supporting recovery from autism.

RECOVERY IN THE 1980s

The definition of recovery in the 1980s was having a 'normal IQ'. Children were tested before and after they received ABA intervention. And the result for many, post ABA, was a 'normal' IQ. These children were placed in regular education in the first grade, but without special assistance. In addition, an independent medical professional authorised to remove a diagnosis would assess the child and confirm a full recovery.

RECOVERY TODAY: ADDITIONAL METHODS OF ASSESSMENT

Recovery today, for Dr Granpeesheh and her team at CARD, means looking at four things: IQ, adaptive functioning, social functioning and language functioning. These, together with executive functioning (i.e. memory, attention and problem solving) and pragmatics of language (being able to have a conversation) are tested to determine recovery. Dr Granpeesheh's team will also assess the child to make sure they're doing well independently at school and making friends. If children still have signs and symptoms of autism, Dr Granpeesheh will *not* classify them as 'fully recovered' until those signs are no longer evident. In a published study on full recovery written by Dr Granpeesheh, all the children assessed as 'normal' were entirely indistinguishable from their peers.

One of the most reliable standardised measures used to determine recovery is the Vineland Adaptive Behaviour Scale, which looks at daily living skills, socialisation and communication, among other things.

In her documentary *Recovered: Journeys through the Autism Spectrum and Back* (2008), Dr Granpeesheh tells the story of four children who recovered from autism. Each child received services, including ABA, from CARD. The documentary shows interviews involving Dr Granpeesheh, the children when they were teenagers, their parents and their therapists. It covers the struggles and triumphs of the journey of recovery, in order to give much-needed knowledge and hope to families of newly diagnosed children that recovery is indeed possible.

EARLY INTERVENTION

Many children *do* completely lose their diagnosis of autism. Often these children will score even higher than their peers on standardised (normal school-entry) tests and will go on to university or college. However, not every child with autism will recover from the condition.

The younger the child and the more hours of ABA they receive early on, the better their chance of recovery. For this reason, I cannot over-emphasise the importance of early intervention; or the need for professionals suspecting autism in a child to refer the parents to an autism expert for the necessary – and potentially life-changing – diagnosis.

According to Dr Granpeesheh, a child's genetic make-up and environmental exposure to toxins early in life may affect the developing brain (and particularly its sensory systems). The ways in which autistic children see, taste and hear things can be totally different from the sensory perceptions of the people around them. Part of the post-recovery treatment means retraining the ways in which they take in and process their environment.

Dr Granpeesheh encourages us to set the bar 'high enough' for each child. If we don't do this, we're accepting less than the child is capable of producing. This is a problem, as autistic children will not, of their own accord, go beyond the limits we set for them. According to Dr Granpeesheh, however, children with autism have no inherent or defined limits. We have to bring out their capabilities by never expecting them to do less than any other child can do.

Fighting for David

For 15 years I've nursed David's autism wounds, becoming quite the medical expert, soothing his pain as best I can and fighting for his functionality. Continuing my unwavering resolve to turn the tide of autism, I can think of nothing but his ultimate cure.

To this end, I've spent hour upon hour upon hour researching biochemistry and studying how the human body works. It's not uncommon for me to stay up really late learning more about the methylation cycle, the mast cell activation of glial cells and mitochondrial dysfunction – all of them part and parcel of the autism diagnosis. And when I wake at 4 am, I pick up where I left off, searching for a way to turn the key to unlock limitless possibility for my son.

Always aware of time and his age, I wrestle the panic that sets in and try to remain focused on the end goal – David's cure.

Martin yearns for the day when he can answer a call from me without having to brace himself for a shock or listen to my automatic reassurance that 'everything's okay'. Eli dreams of attending a top medical school. Exposed to his parents' discussions of microbiology in the kitchen and looking further than the symptoms to find a cure for David, Eli has already started to plan his future attack on autism. I have no doubt that he will be continuing the rescue operation beyond our lifetime.

There has to be a cure

I'm confident that somewhere and somehow the universe holds the answer: I simply need to reach out and grab it. It may be lying hidden in the bowels of the earth. It may be sitting on top of a shooting star or in an ice crevice tucked away at the North Pole. Wherever it is and whatever it takes, I'm determined to find it.

I need to keep looking and digging. Like a mathematician solving complex maths equations, I continue to study and delve into the cellular level of David's autism, breaking down every component one by one. As night settles in and the peacefulness of evening envelops me, I know I'm close …

Our journey through uncharted terrain is ongoing – with many days when I feel saddened, disheartened and even defeated by the powerful force that keeps David from us. I constantly battle the stress and anxiety that goes hand in hand with autism. Not daring to venture too far from my phone in case of an emergency and tracking every step he takes. Trying to push out the deep feelings of worry and the sense of loss; and replacing them with action and positive thoughts.

Changing the medical mindset

I call on all health professionals in this country and elsewhere to open their minds and embrace the many new areas of research and evidence-based treatments in this field. Autism has been so misunderstood for so many years … The time has come for change!

This is especially needed because of the significant growth in the number of children diagnosed with autism – a growth that cannot be explained merely through the improved diagnosis of this condition in the past decades. Autism has hit our planet like a raging tsunami – out of control, demonstrating nature's fury. But where are the South African doctors looking for the explosive forces behind the autism tsunami?

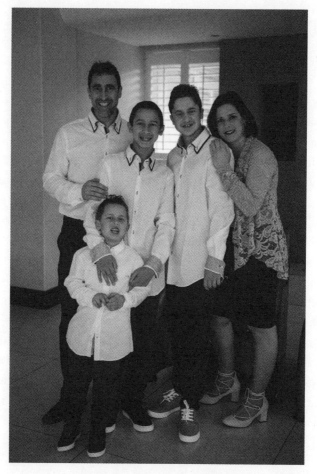

The indomitable Gerschlowitz family

Psychiatric medication can no longer be accepted as a valid first line of treatment for children with autism in South Africa. Our situation, which includes a citizenry mostly uneducated about autism and ways of treating it, is calling out for a medical community that thinks about the condition in a much more enlightened and holistic manner. Medical doctors, psychologists, psychiatrists, occupational therapists, speech therapists, nutritionists, teachers and other school staff: the evidence concerning treatment options and in support of autism recovery is simply undeniable.

With all the knowledge on autism now at our disposal, what might once have been regarded as a doctor's careless and heartless attitude to diagnosing autism in a child might today be seen as medical negligence. Help is at hand, and 'Goodbye and good luck' no longer quite cuts it.

A happy ending for every autistic child

There's nothing more my heart desires than to restore health and functionality to David and every autistic child who walks through our doors at The Star Academy. We know this is possible. *Aaron is the proof that early intervention sets the stage for full recovery.*

Just the other day I told Martin that I still haven't given up hope that one day David will do things that remain unimaginable to us. We have to conquer his limitations no matter the cost. Martin initially gave me a look that may have said 'crazy woman' but needed little convincing to go along with my hopeful outlook. No day will end, no sun will set, without us searching for David's cure. I know it's out there.

DIAGNOSING AUTISM IN YOUNG CHILDREN

THE RED FLAGS OF AUTISM IN A DEVELOPING CHILD

It's important for parents, teachers and other people responsible for looking after children on a daily basis to be familiar with the typical developmental milestones all children should be reaching; and to learn about the early signs of autism.

The following checklist of autism **red flags** may indicate that a child is at risk of being diagnosed with autism. In some children, the early signs of autism may be observed by 12 months or even earlier. This is particularly important to note because, until very recently in South Africa, it was believed that you could diagnose autism only from three years of age.

If a child presents with any of the following, please don't delay further investigation, and see a doctor or paediatrician:

❑ Lack of eye contact
❑ Not responding appropriately to greetings or when their name is called
❑ Not engaging in pretend play
❑ Preferring to play alone
❑ Not playing peek-a-boo by eight months
❑ Not babbling by 12 months
❑ No back-and-forth gestures such as pointing or showing by 12 months
❑ No imitative behaviour such as waving bye-bye by 12 months

- ❏ No words by 16 months
- ❏ No meaningful, two-word phrases (not including imitating or repeating) by 24 months
- ❏ Any loss of speech at any age
- ❏ Losing previously acquired skills at any age
- ❏ No sharing of enjoyment or interest
- ❏ Becoming distressed by minor changes in routines
- ❏ Performing repetitive movements such as hand flapping or rocking
- ❏ Playing with toys in unusual ways, for example by spinning them or lining them up
- ❏ Having unusually strong attachments to particular objects
- ❏ Limiting conversations to very specific topics
- ❏ Exhibiting oversensitivity to sounds or textures
- ❏ Being a picky eater
- ❏ Experiencing plateaus or delays in skills development
- ❏ Displaying challenging behaviours such as aggression, tantrums and self-injury
- ❏ Appearing to be in their own world
- ❏ Not following any, or following too few, receptive instructions
- ❏ Repetitive movements with objects or posturing of body, arms, hands or fingers
- ❏ Being hyperactive
- ❏ Being unable to sustain their attention compared to their peers

THE MODIFIED CHECKLIST FOR AUTISM IN TODDLERS, REVISED (M-CHAT-R)

This checklist is a free, validated screening tool of 20 questions that assesses a child's risk of autism. If you have concerns about your child's development, tick the aspect(s) you see as concerning and contact your doctor or paediatrician. If you're a teacher and have noticed possible signs of autism in a child, express your concerns tactfully yet immediately to the child's parents. Show them the checklist and what you've ticked as concerning, and advise them to take the list to a doctor or a paediatrician.

Please answer questions to reflect your child's usual behaviours. If the behaviour is rare (for example, you've seen it only once or twice), answer as if the child has not acquired the behaviour.

1. If you point at something across the room, does your child look at it? *(For example, if you point at a toy or an animal, does your child look at the toy or animal?)* YES / NO

2. Have you ever wondered if your child might be deaf? *YES / NO*

3. Does your child play pretend or make-believe? *(For example, pretend to drink from an empty cup, pretend to talk on a phone, or pretend to feed a doll or stuffed animal?)* YES / NO

4. Does your child like climbing on things? *(For example, furniture, playground equipment, or stairs)* YES / NO

5. Does your child make unusual finger movements near his or her eyes? *(For example, does your child wiggle his or her fingers close to his or her eyes?)* YES / NO

6. Does your child point with one finger to ask for something or to get help? *(For example, pointing to a snack or toy that is out of reach)* YES / NO

7. Does your child point with one finger to show you something interesting? *(For example, pointing to an airplane in the sky or a big truck in the road)* YES / NO

8. Is your child interested in other children? *(For example, does your child watch other children, smile at them, or go to them?)* YES / NO

9. Does your child show you things by bringing them to you or holding them up for you to see – not to get help, but just to share? *(For example, showing you a flower, a stuffed animal, or a toy truck)* YES / NO

10. Does your child respond when you call his or her name? *(For example, does he or she look up, talk or babble, or stop what he or she is doing when you call his or her name?)* YES / NO

11. When you smile at your child, does he or she smile back at you? *YES / NO*

12. Does your child get upset by everyday noises? *(For example, does your child scream or cry at noises such as that made by a vacuum cleaner, or loud music?) YES / NO*

13. Does your child walk? *YES / NO*

14. Does your child look you in the eye when you are talking to him or her, playing with him or her, or dressing him or her? *YES / NO*

15. Does your child try to copy what you do? *(For example, wave bye-bye, clap, or make a funny noise when you do) YES / NO*

16. If you turn your head to look at something, does your child look around to see what you are looking at? *YES / NO*

17. Does your child try to get you to watch him or her? *(For example, does your child look at you for praise, or say 'look' or 'watch me'?) YES / NO*

18. Does your child understand when you tell him or her to do something? *(For example, if you don't point, can your child understand 'put the book on the chair' or 'bring me the blanket'?) YES / NO*

19. If something new happens, does your child look at your face to see how you feel about it? *(For example, if he or she hears a strange or funny noise, or sees a new toy, will he or she look at your face?) YES / NO*

20. Does your child like movement activities? *(For example, being swung or bounced on your knee) YES / NO*

Source: Robins D, Fein D & Barton M (1999): *Modified Checklist for Autism in Toddlers, Revised (M-CHAT-R)*, available at https://www.autismspeaks.org/screen-your-child, accessed 10 April 2019

THE AUTISM SPECTRUM

In 2013, the American Psychiatric Association released the fifth edition of its *Diagnostic and Statistical Manual of Mental Disorders* (DSM-5). The handbook is used by healthcare professionals in the United States and much of the world as the authoritative guide to the diagnosis of autism. The DSM-5 replaced the DSM-4 which placed autism into categories including Pervasive Developmental Disorder (PDD), Pervasive Developmental Disorder Not Otherwise Specified (PDD NOS) and Asperger's. With the new DSM-5 these categories have all been merged, and there is now one diagnosis called Autism Spectrum Disorder.

Understanding ASD in terms of the diagnostic criteria laid out in the DSM-5 is depicted below:

Autism Spectrum Disorder: Diagnostic Criteria

A. Persistent deficits in social communication and social interaction across multiple contexts, as manifested by the following, currently or by history (examples are illustrative, not exhaustive; see text):
   1. Deficits in social-emotional reciprocity, ranging, for example, from abnormal social approach and failure of normal back-and-forth conversation; to reduced sharing of interests, emotions, or affect; to failure to initiate or respond to social interactions.
   2. Deficits in nonverbal communicative behaviours used for social

interaction, ranging, for example, from poorly integrated verbal and nonverbal communication; to abnormalities in eye contact and body language or deficits in understanding and use of gestures; to a total lack of facial expressions and nonverbal communication.

3. Deficits in developing, maintaining, and understanding relationships, ranging, for example, from difficulties adjusting behaviour to suit various social contexts; to difficulties in sharing imaginative play or in making friends; to absence of interest in peers.

Specify current severity: Severity is based on social-communication impairments and restricted repetitive patterns of behaviour. (See table on page 311.)

B. Restricted, repetitive patterns of behaviour, interests, or activities, as manifested by at least two of the following, currently or by history (examples are illustrative, not exhaustive; see text):

1. Stereotyped or repetitive motor movements, use of objects, or speech (e.g. simple motor stereotypes, lining up toys or flipping objects, echolalia, idiosyncratic phrases).

2. Insistence on sameness, inflexible adherence to routines, or ritualised patterns of verbal or nonverbal behaviour (e.g. extreme distress at small changes, difficulties with transitions, rigid thinking patterns, greeting rituals, need to take same route or eat same food every day).

3. Highly restricted, fixated interests that are abnormal in intensity or focus (e.g. strong attachment to or preoccupation with unusual objects, excessively circumscribed or persevering interest).

4. Hyper- or hypo-reactivity to sensory input or unusual interests in sensory aspects of the environment (e.g. apparent indifference to pain/temperature, adverse response to specific sounds or textures, excessive smelling or touching of objects, visual fascination with lights or movement).

Specify current severity: Severity is based on social-communication impairments and restricted, repetitive patterns of behaviour. (See table.)

C. Symptoms must be present in the early developmental period (but may not become fully manifest until social demands exceed limited capacities or may be masked by learned strategies in later life).

D. Symptoms cause clinically significant impairment in social, occupational, or other important areas of current functioning.

E. These disturbances are not better explained by intellectual disability (intellectual-developmental disorder) or global developmental delay. Intellectual disability and ASD frequently co-occur; to make co-morbid diagnoses of ASD and intellectual disability, social communication should be below that expected for general developmental level.

Note: Individuals with a well-established DSM-4 diagnosis of autistic disorder, Asperger's disorder, or PDD not otherwise specified should be given the diagnosis of ASD. Individuals who have marked deficits in social communication, but whose symptoms do not otherwise meet criteria for ASD, should be evaluated for social (pragmatic) communication disorder.

Specify if:
❑ With or without accompanying intellectual impairment
❑ With or without accompanying language impairment
❑ Associated with a known medical or genetic condition or environmental factor (Coding note: Use additional code to identify the associated medical or genetic condition.)
❑ Associated with another neurodevelopmental, mental, or behavioural disorder
(Coding note: Use additional code[s] to identify the associated neurodevelopmental, mental, or behavioural disorder[s].)
❑ With catatonia

SEVERITY LEVELS FOR AUTISM SPECTRUM DISORDER		
Severity level	Social communication	Restricted, repetitive behaviours
Level 3 'Requiring very substantial support'	Level 2 'Requiring substantial support'	Level 1 'Requiring support'
Severe deficits in verbal and nonverbal social-communication skills cause severe impairments in functioning, very limited initiation of social interactions, and minimal response to social overtures from others. For example, a person with few words of intelligible speech who rarely initiates interaction and, when he or she does, makes unusual approaches to meet needs only and responds to only very direct social approaches. Inflexibility of behaviour, extreme difficulty coping with change, or other restricted/ repetitive behaviours markedly interfere with functioning in all spheres. Great distress/difficulty changing focus or action.	Marked deficits in verbal and nonverbal social-communication skills; social impairments apparent even with supports in place; limited initiation of social interactions; and reduced or abnormal responses to social overtures from others. For example, a person who speaks simple sentences, whose interaction is limited to narrow special interests, and who has markedly odd nonverbal communication. Inflexibility of behaviour, difficulty coping with change, or other restricted/repetitive behaviours appear frequently enough to be obvious to the casual observer and interfere with functioning in a variety of contexts. Distress and/or difficulty changing focus or action.	Without supports in place, deficits in social communication cause noticeable impairments. Difficulty initiating social interactions, and clear examples of atypical or unsuccessful response to social overtures of others. May appear to have decreased interest in social interactions. For example, a person who is able to speak in full sentences and engages in communication but whose to-and-fro conversation with others fails, and whose attempts to make friends are odd and typically unsuccessful. Inflexibility of behaviour causes significant interference with functioning in one or more contexts. Difficulty switching between activities. Problems of organisation and planning hamper independence.

Social (Pragmatic) Communication Disorder: Diagnostic Criteria

A. Persistent difficulties in the social use of verbal and nonverbal communication as manifested by all of the following:

 1. Deficits in using communication for social purposes, such as greeting and sharing information, in a manner that is appropriate for the social context.

 2. Impairment of the ability to change communication to match context or the needs of the listener, such as speaking differently in a classroom than on the playground, talking differently to a child than to an adult, and avoiding use of overly formal language.

 3. Difficulties following rules for conversation and storytelling, such as taking turns in conversation, rephrasing when misunderstood, and knowing how to use verbal and nonverbal signals to regulate interaction.

 4. Difficulties understanding what is not explicitly stated (e.g. making inferences) and nonliteral or ambiguous meanings of language (e.g. idioms, humour, metaphors, multiple meanings that depend on the context for interpretation).

B. The deficits result in functional limitations in effective communication, social participation, social relationships, academic achievement, or occupational performance, individually or in combination.

C. The onset of the symptoms is in the early developmental period (but deficits may not become fully manifest until social communication demands exceed limited capacities).

D. The symptoms are not attributable to another medical or neurological condition or to low abilities in the domains of word structure and grammar, and are not better explained by ASD, intellectual disability (intellectual-developmental disorder), global developmental delay, of another mental disorder.

Source: American Psychiatric Association, Fifth Edition (2013): *Diagnostic and Statistical Manual of Mental Disorders (DSM-5)*, available at https://www.autismspeaks.org/dsm-5-criteria, accessed 10 April 2019

DEBUNKING MYTHS AROUND AUTISM SPECTRUM DISORDER

Children with an ASD have a variety of symptoms, presenting them in different ways and to different degrees. Although ASD is often surrounded by stereotypical misconceptions and myths, each case is unique, requiring a tailor-made programme addressing each child's particular needs and specific skill deficits. Here are the top six myths about autism.

MYTH 1: THERE IS NO CURE

Truth: There are two key interventions which address an autism diagnosis: Applied Behaviour Analysis (ABA) and biomedical treatment. ABA is evidence-based treatment for children with autism and a medical neccessity. Bio-medical treatment includes treating the underlying causes of autism such as inflammation, immune dysregulation, viral/fungal/bacterial infections, impaired detoxification, food allergies, nutrient deficiencies and impaired methylation. Evidence-based medicine proves that autism can be a treatable medical illness.

MYTH 2: AUTISM IS A LIFELONG DISORDER

Truth: Autism need not be a lifelong disorder. According to the Center for Disease Control and Prevention, research shows that early intervention treatment from birth to 36 months can greatly improve a child's development. Autism is treatable and recovery possible.

MYTH 3: PEOPLE WITH AUTISM SHOULD BE PLACED IN A SPECIAL-NEEDS SCHOOL

Truth: A one-size-fits-all approach doesn't work because each child has a unique manifestation of autism. Every person with autism must be treated and assessed on an individual basis. An Individualised Education Plan (IEP) should be designed for each child.

MYTH 4: ALL PEOPLE WITH AUTISM HAVE THE SAME SKILLS AND DIFFICULTIES

Truth: While people with ASD have certain overlapping symptoms such as repetitive behaviours, challenges with social interaction and sensory processing, each child on the spectrum has unique interests, deficits and their own particular weaknesses, strengths and abilities.

MYTH 5: CHILDREN WITH AUTISM CANNOT FORM CONNECTIONS WITH OTHERS

Truth: Children with autism may not always perceive the subtleties of body language or the nuance of tone in a voice, which means they may not detect sadness or sarcasm. However, this doesn't stop them from enjoying fulfilling relationships with parents, siblings, spouses and children. It does mean, however, that they can experience challenges in navigating social relationships and understanding social cues.

MYTH 6: CHILDREN WITH AUTISM CANNOT SPEAK

Truth: Although some children with autism may be nonverbal or may have delayed speech, there are other children whose speech is well developed. Delayed speech can be addressed by therapies such as ABA and PROMPT. Children who are nonverbal can be supported by speech-augmentation devices which facilitate communication, and vocal productions can always be worked on and improved.

Source: The Star Academy